Breathwork
for
Pregnancy

Breathwork for Pregnancy

How to Find Calm throughout the Four Trimesters

CAROLYN COWAN

Zeitgeist • New York

Published in the United States by Zeitgeist, an imprint of Zeitgeist™,
a division of Penguin Random House LLC, New York.
zeitgeistpublishing.com

Zeitgeist™ is a trademark of Penguin Random House LLC
ISBN: 9780593886526
Ebook ISBN: 9780593886489

Originally published as *Breathing for Pregnancy* in paperback in Great Britain by Vermilion,
an imprint of Ebury Publishing, a division of Penguin Random House Ltd., London, in
2023. Ebury is part of the Penguin Random House group of companies.

Cover design by Holly Ovenden
Cover photo by Carolyn Cowan

Printed in the United States of America
1st Printing

First United States Edition

*To all mothers bringing forth children
who will create change in the world.*

CONTENTS

Introduction

Let us sit down together under this wonderful, generous, patient old oak tree and discuss. Get comfortable. I have brought a blanket and a small pillow for you to sit on.

You are here, we meet, because you are pregnant.

Being with child is a miraculous process, but it is also an intensely internal experience, physically and emotionally, deeply rooted in our survival instincts: we have an urge to reproduce, to improve the human race. The hormonal changes that take place from the moment of conception are rooted in our primal instincts to create safety, to nest, to make a safe place in which to bring up the child, and to protect ourselves and the child during and after the gestation process.

Pregnancy and beyond can take myriad different forms, and each pregnancy, every child born, is unique. There are so many ways in which the process can unfold, grow and emerge from within us and for all those around us.

For many, getting pregnant is heavenly bliss: the 40 weeks are divine and the birth experience is a net of professional safety around us, as we trust the midwives, the doctors and the guided process. For others it might be a magical home experience with a birthing pool and a midwife all to yourself.

Picking up this book, you may be absolutely fabulously well, feeling great, blossoming into pregnancy, loving every moment of this time and just wanting to enjoy breathwork as a way to be present and peaceful. If this is you, then throughout this book I will talk you through the many ways in which you can work with your mind and body to stay relaxed and calm using the breath.

For some, discovering they are pregnant can be initially overwhelming, unexpected, even terrifying. It may be all that you ever longed for and, even so, that moment of knowing it is real, that the embryo is within you and growing, can open up so many previously unthought processes, feelings and changes to your reality.

Holding the pregnancy for 40 weeks as your body meets the growing embryo's demands, the changes to your physicality and thoughts, and, week by week, counting down toward labor can feel like the last great voyage into the unknown. *Who will this child be? Who am I creating? Who are we creating?* These are all lovely questions that are perfectly normal to ask at this time. You will find that you will adapt, settle into the 40 weeks and find your particular rhythm, and your fears and overwhelm will subside.

You may also be here because you want me, and the breathwork and stretching I will teach you, to help you manage anxious thinking, worrying thoughts, deep fears. I cannot stop these thoughts and feelings forever; however, what you will learn in these pages is how to calm yourself down. The wonderful news is that you have the ability to change how you think and feel, and the fastest way for that to happen is through movement and the breath.

"Attunement" describes this ability to become aware of when your nervous system is in the stress response. You will learn to attune to your own state of being, notice if it is not serving you, change how you feel and, in this action and choice, become present and gentle. This will then be felt by all those around and within you, and in turn they will become calm, too.

This book is about finding calm in pregnancy through "conscious breathing" in the first three trimesters—the gestation period, while the child (or children) grows within you—and the fourth trimester, the postnatal phase.

WHAT IS CONSCIOUS BREATHING?

To breathe consciously is to take over, when you choose, the body's unconscious breath patterns. These can be easily understood by noticing how many times you breathe in a minute. There is an ideal breath length, for both the inhale and the exhale, for being present—right here, right now—and in this conscious breath pattern your mind and body are safe enough for all functions—mind, heart rate and hormonal flow—to be in their optimal state.

As you will learn in these pages, this optimal state of being has a profound impact on the child both within and, post-labor, outside your body. In Chapter 5 I will take you through breaths that invite you to breathe more slowly and take you into deeper states of stillness, presence and calm.

Set a timer on your phone for one minute. Without judging yourself or trying to do it perfectly, sit up and count each inhale and exhale until the timer goes off.

You may be calm, peaceful and gentle when you try this and arrive at around ten breaths per minute, or perhaps fewer. Try again when you notice you feel stressed or rushed or have just had a moment with social media or the news. You may find that, in that minute of counting your breaths, you breathe faster; the count may be closer to 16 breaths per minute. This is OK; it is not bad or wrong but a perfect example of *unconscious* breathing. Your mind and body will have been mobilized by the situation so, in response to your thoughts, your unconscious breath pattern will have automatically sped up.

Over the course of reading this book and the different scenarios I will invite you into, you will learn how to notice your unconscious breathing and change over to conscious breathing. You will also learn the breath length you are aiming for.

I want to bring you to a good understanding of why you should breathe consciously, particularly in pregnancy, without blinding you with science at an already complex time. We will explore how your body and mind work together, and I will share with you the best of breathwork practice to facilitate your need for a kind space in which to find yourself, for yourself, by yourself, as a pregnant woman, no matter what your pregnancy journey looks like.

Conscious breathing is a highly accessible practice and has so many benefits in pregnancy:

- The act of breathing deeply and slowly sends more oxygen to the growing fetus and improves your whole system, changing hormonal flow and thus calming the baby, too.
- Conscious breathing brings a sense of awareness and—particularly in the afterglow, when I ask that you take two minutes to be still, calm and gentle—it is an opportunity to connect deeply to the child within you.
- You will find that you have more energy for your day and your mood will be good.
- Breathwork facilitates better sleep. Finding calm also helps to manage blood pressure.

- It is a personal practice, and my hope is that you will find this for yourself by making space in your day and taking downtime away from screens and other stressors.
- Breathwork in pregnancy allows you to be calm and centered, making a very real difference to the child inside you, your sense of self and how much you can enjoy being pregnant.

Just a few minutes of conscious breathing makes a big difference to the mind and body.

You may have already done a lot of breathwork, particularly if you like to practice yoga. Many yogic forms include similar breathing practices—particularly the type I teach, Kundalini Global—but nowhere else is there a specific adaptation of these techniques to allow for the rapidly changing body that you find yourself in charge of as a pregnant woman. What we will do here is unique, well researched and taught in the thousands of Kundalini Global classes and yoga teacher training courses that I run.

I have also included a specific chapter on stretching in this book (Chapter 4). Stretching and sitting in silence is a work of building intimacy with yourself. Over time, you will begin to notice that it becomes easier to bear yourself, by yourself, for yourself. This will, in turn, change how you experience yourself in your daily life and in personal interactions. These practices are the foundations for good boundaries and they foster the ability to recognize when self-care is more useful than being reactive.

Conscious breathing combined with stretching is yours—entirely yours. It is a superpower, a magical portal into transformation and change. It is a glorious practice that gives you agency over yourself. My hope is that you will take on a personal daily practice in your pregnancy that will serve you for the rest of your life.

Throughout your pregnancy and into the postnatal period, you will be able to share this ability to manage and hold your emotional being with the next generation. This is the amazing gift of all that we will be doing together. This is work that you will do for yourself but that your children, your family and all those around you can also benefit from.

WHO AM I?

My task is to show you how to change how you feel, to assist you in beginning to trust the process you are going through and to teach you that, at any time, you can simply, quietly and all by yourself change how you feel. This is what I do; it is my job. You could even say that this is who I am: the breath teacher.

I know how to do this, how to teach you, because I have been a version of who you are now. I was a pregnant woman, a while ago now. My children are now adults, but for me, getting pregnant, going through multiple losses and being in an unhappy relationship combined with having a "tall dark history" made my own experiences of being pregnant quite stressful.

(A tall dark history is my euphemism for the word trauma. "Tall dark history" allows for all manner of events to have been there in the past, without them having to also be in the present.)

I was overwhelmed, scared and, at times, very difficult to be with. As I landed in the postnatal phase, depression and overwhelm took hold and I knew I needed tools to cope. I needed to change my relationship to my fears, my stress and my anxiety.

At that time I worked alone to find a way through, to change the way I felt, and the breath came to me, almost as gently as you now find me. Little by little, I learned to work with, not against, my stress system—to stretch and, from there, to consciously breathe.

This led me to being able to calm myself, to stay relaxed and to be present. The rest is history—herstory. Both my children and our relational processes, informed by my ability to attune to myself and find calm, have benefited from my emotional growth.

Alongside and because of this life-changing awareness, I trained to be a psychotherapist and a yoga teacher, specializing in the pre- and postnatal phases. I have worked with the issues around making babies for almost three decades now.

As you read about and begin to practice the many concepts, tools and breaths in this book, perhaps you could allow me to be a friend who has their hand on your back. A mentor, walking beside you. Someone who is "on your side."

I AM NOT A DOCTOR

I cannot define your route through pregnancy and beyond. I wish to be, in a writerly way, someone who sees you, can speak to you and with you, and can help you to move through this time in your life with more ease than you had before you picked up this book. But I am not a guru. Not a doctor. Not a midwife. Not an obstetrician. Please remember that. I am your breath teacher.

In my experience of being a teacher, I have found that it can be easy for those I teach to assume I know far more than I do, that somehow the very lovely experiences we can have together will negate or replace medical advice, that you can give all responsibility to me. Yet medical intervention might be needed for some issues.

I have good boundaries; I know when medical advice needs to come to the fore. If I know there are edges to my usefulness, I will name them.

HOW TO USE THIS BOOK

As a therapist I understand the link between mind and body, stressful thoughts and feelings, and how we are affected by and can affect others. How we think profoundly impacts how we feel. When you are upbeat, smiling, laughing, full of the joys of pregnancy, your physical body is in tune with this mindset. In daily life much can knock us out of this centered place and, when our mind and thoughts become constricted, repetitive or judgmental of ourselves or others, our body changes accordingly. This is why I have focused Part 1 of this book on understanding how the stress system works, how it is activated and how to release it. The knowledge I share in these specific chapters will assist you in learning how to use the power of the breath and stretching to find calm.

In Part 2 I bring you the stretches and the breaths. As a breathwork and yoga teacher, my learning has been deeply rooted in how the mind and body can be profoundly altered by conscious breathing and specific stretching movements, prior to breathwork, which bring their own benefits to the mind–body axis, and add depth to the effects of conscious breathing.

In Chapter 4 you will learn to stretch before breathing to make it easier for you to be calm and centered. I will encourage you to understand how to stretch to get the most from the breathing options, alongside helping you to be comfortable in the constantly changing form that is a pregnant body. I encourage you to use props to help you get confident with the movements you can do so that you can make the most of your commitment to a regular practice (see page 10).

You can stretch without breathing afterward, just for the sheer pleasure of the release and equally, you can breathe consciously without stretching. What I can tell you, though, is that the two work together beautifully.

I have dedicated a whole chapter—Chapter 5—to gifting you a variety of breaths to use in pregnancy and beyond. I have been teaching these techniques for 25 years at the time of writing, and I am in love with each of the breaths I have chosen to include for you. Each has its own personality, its own character, if you will, and they individually bring you to different states of being, surprisingly quickly.

In all the teaching I have done, I have noticed that it is really easy to limit a breath to a specific issue or desire, but this closes off so much potential. Just because you have tried one breath and found it useful for morning sickness, like "The Straw Breath" (page 150), that does not mean you cannot also use it if you want to relax before bed or take some time when you are overwhelmed. The breaths all work for different people in different ways. My hope is that you will play with them, over time, in a variety of contexts. This way you will build agency for yourself, to know which breaths work best for you, when and where.

Part 3 explores each trimester individually, focusing on the challenges you may face and the individual breathwork and stretches that will support you in your journey.

It may be that you want to skip all the chapters leading up to the breathwork and, of course, you are free to do so, but in the decades of teaching these techniques I have become aware that understanding how the stress system works, and how the breath changes it, is extremely helpful. The pregnant body is a wonder of the first order, with myriad different changes taking place. I am a fan of understanding why you are taking on these practices in order to better facilitate the experience. This understanding has a positive impact on the experience of stretching and sitting to practice. Holding the knowledge I will share opens you up to all that is available to you in the breaths. Of course, I suggest reading it all.

My writing style is gentle, and each chapter opens with some reflections, written as if I were in the midst of a moment with you. It may be a stressful or challenging moment that I will use to help illustrate what I want you to know, to understand how your mind, body and feelings are linked and to show you how much you can do to turn this to your and your baby's advantage by taking over your sensations of stress through these practices.

This is a deep intimacy, a generous space that we can drop into together. You may read a section and think, *That is not me, I cannot imagine you,* but I will do my best to create a scene, a feeling that you can perhaps identify with—so could you allow the details to be imperfect but in the right area? This will open up the different breaths for you to try in various states of being, as well as just for the sheer pleasure of conscious breathwork.

PROPS ARE YOUR FRIEND

You may have previously practiced a form of yoga that eschewed any kind of assistance in terms of sitting, standing or stretching. If this is the case, I invite you now to explore a landscape of adjustments to facilitate your changing and, later, recovering body.

If you can purchase or borrow the few key items listed below, they will be an investment in this entire experience.

If you are discovering yourself—body and mind—through this book, please do take a look at everything that is described here. It may be that in early pregnancy your body is compliant to the stretches, needing little or no support from props, but over the months you'll find that your needs will change.

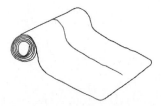

A yoga mat

The ritualistic action of rolling out the mat will make your practice habitual. Each time you unfurl this mat, you are choosing to make and take time for yourself, to give yourself back to yourself. You can do this even if, through pregnancy, you place a chair on top of the mat rather than getting down on the floor. The yoga mat also provides non-slip support for stretches, standing or seated.

I would avoid using a foam mat. Even though they are cheaper by far than a high-quality yoga mat that could cost you $75–100, they are profoundly annoying because they dent and will not lie flat, are easily damaged and take up a lot more space in their stubborn unwieldiness. A foam mat robustly refuses to play nicely. You can use a towel instead of purchasing a mat, but please be aware that it will not provide a stable surface.

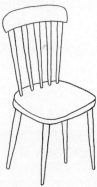

An upright chair with good stability

A kitchen or dining chair is a good option. Sit with your spine straight, tailbone untucked, rather than leaning back into the chair.

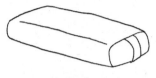

A bolster

A bolster is a wide, low, firm support, either for your pelvis, to raise the hips higher than the knees, or for tight hamstrings, to help the tension in the back of your legs when they are straight, either standing or sitting wide-legged. You can use a sofa cushion or a pillow instead. A large, folded blanket also works well.

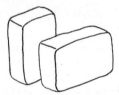

Two brick-shaped blocks

Blocks are good for propping up stiff knees, and if tight hamstrings make it uncomfortable to sit with your legs out straight, they can be used flat beneath each knee when sitting on the bolster. Postnatally, one block is comfortable under the head for post-stretch or breathwork relaxation. Make sure your blocks are cork (not foam or wood).

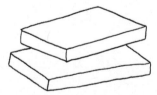

A flat, high-density foam block

This helps to give a small lift to the pelvis when seated and can assist in forward folds in standing postures, taking the pressure off the lower back and artificially raising the floor in front of you for your hands to rest upon. You can use a couple of large books instead.

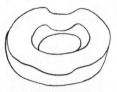

A donut pillow

If you have postnatal pain or discomfort in the labial area and/or anus, then this ring of cushioning will help you sit anywhere.

A yoga strap

This is a long, cotton webbing strap with a pinch buckle, which means it can be adjusted to hold itself in different lengths. It is most often used to facilitate stretching out. A cotton scarf is an easy replacement here.

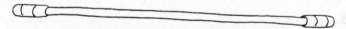

A broom handle or similar pole

I know it sounds odd, but this can come in very handy for helping you get up from the floor, rather than heaving yourself up. In standing postures the pole gives balance.

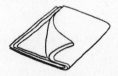

A blanket or shawl

In the chill of the dawn light, when sitting to breathe, post-stretching, during breathwork or in relaxation, having a soft shawl around your shoulders or over your whole body is a lovely thing.

Two cushions or bed pillows

Cushions help with lying on your left side in relaxation during the last few weeks of gestation. Use one folded between the knees to ease the pelvis, and the other under the higher elbow to lift pressure off the breasts. Add a brick block or a thick book beneath your head to straighten the spine and this becomes a comfortable resting position. Pillows are also lovely under the head if you are relaxing with a bolster under your knees.

DO YOUR COMFORTABLE BEST

You can begin working with this book at any stage in your pregnancy journey. You can do the breathwork that is included for pregnancy at any time during gestation (the breaths only suitable post-birth are clearly labeled as such).

Later in the book we will look at taking on a daily practice. If you're new to breathwork, I would suggest that you begin by choosing a stretch or a breath and reading through the explanation a few times. Try it out for a couple of rounds and then get comfortable and set a timer for one minute. This is a good way to get started and feel more confident.

If you feel you are ready to try for longer, three minutes is a good practice time and allows you to become aware of how you respond to the transformations that conscious stretching and breathing practices bring to you. Take this on for three minutes per day, perhaps for a week to get familiar with it. Set aside enough time to get comfortable (choose some music if you would like) and to sit, in stillness, for a few minutes afterward.

If something doesn't feel right—in the unlikely event that you feel lightheaded, for example—please slow down your practice and mention your experience to your midwife and/or doctor.

Be careful not to stand up too quickly after sitting for a long period of time; take it slowly and gently and if you have high blood pressure notice if this feels wrong or uncomfortable.

It is easy to think that you need to be perfect and that you must instantly master breathwork. This is not true. There will be interruptions, from other people, your own mind, the child inside kicking, a relentless need to pee. So many people, places and things can trip up your drive for perfection.

You are with me so I can teach you. Learning is a process; it takes time. There will be instant responses, awarenesses and changes in your mind and body—instant payoff! But as you become more familiar with the various practices in this book, they will begin to resonate differently. This unfolding never stops. It is a big part of the learning, particularly in how you will become more able to recognize the experiences of stillness, gentleness and peace.

What I ask is that you always do your comfortable best. You can facilitate this by limiting distractions where you can, like your phone. Of course, you may choose to use your phone as a timer, but if you do, put it on silent and turn it face down so you will not see it light up with notifications—these create an imperative to action, and we are stretching and breathing for stillness.

There are so many ways that the techniques in this book can help to create time, space and calm around and within you. Over the coming chapters, we will look at different emotions and situations that may arise in which you can choose to take a moment, stretch the tension out and take a breath break. When you do this you will facilitate seeing and feeling more clearly.

YOUR PREGNANT IDENTITY

Were you gifted this book? Perhaps by your partner? Maybe you have had a breath practice for a while and wish to continue with breaths appropriate to what you are going through now. Or perhaps the title called out to you from a bookshelf and here we are.

I want to welcome you on this journey by saying that, however you found yourself reaching for this book, please know that I am highly respectful of all the different iterations of fertility, pregnancy, birth and parenting.

My own experience of being pregnant was that I felt as though so much of my identity was lost, swept under my bump. My career, interests, desire to dance, thoughts, sense of humor, politics and needs sometimes felt as though they were lost in the expectations of others, alongside my swiftly changing body.

I would like to say, before we begin the journey through this book as companions, that I walk with *all* of you, not just the you in your pregnant identity. Your identity as a person is not lost.

When I work as a therapist, I go on adventures that are not dissimilar to the one we are about to begin, with an array of interesting, unique and individual humans. I get to know each person well—as well as they allow me to—and our dialogue becomes as unique as they are. The intimacy we create is important to the work, and so, in writing this book, I reflected enormously on how we could develop that intimacy between us, too.

You will notice that I address you as my companion. *You.*

You are an original. In that, you are complex. I aim to represent a rich tapestry made up of individual pregnant experiences, and so it is unlikely that I will get *you*, your feelings, thoughts, preferences and responses perfectly every time.

I cannot think, on any level, that I know you or your circumstances—whether you have a partner, previous children, stepkids or how you arrived at being pregnant. I know nothing, but I aim to be inclusive and encompassing in all the ways I know how to be.

If you are someone who does not sit within expected cultural, religious or gender roles, believe me when I say I understand. If I could write a book that reflected the richness of humanity, I would. As that is not possible in a landscape that is moving rapidly in regards to identity, I have made the decision to use the word "woman" to best represent those who will be choosing to walk with me through these pages.

I sit beside you, our arms close. I am here, with you, through all the different phases of your pregnancy and into the postnatal phase.

Let's take a moment; lean back with me against this beautiful tree. Feel the sun on your skin and allow all the muscles of your face to relax. Become soft. Take your hand off your phone. Just let the light, the birdsong and this moment between us be all that there is, right now.

PART 1

Understanding the Stress Response

Chapter 1

The Activated
Stress System

I am making cups of tea for us, hearing you on the phone to a friend talking about a comment someone made when you announced you were pregnant.

"She said what?!"… And then … "No! You cannot be serious!"

I sit down to join you at the kitchen table. It is a lovely sunny winter's day and the low light glances across the room. Outside, the sky is a crisp blue and there is frost in the garden.

You slam down your phone and huff. In a further fit of anger you push it away, but then you pick it up again to light up the screen and check for any messages that might have silently crept in.

You are indignant, furious, incandescent even. I love that word. "Do you know what it means?" I ask you. No, it seems not, as you do not answer. It means ablaze with fury.

What a perfect invitation for you to tell me all about it now.

Sitting back with your arms folded, you glare at me and say, "What?"

"Nothing." I smile and drink my tea.

You are frowning, shoulders hunched, breathing fast. "How can you be so calm?" you demand, irritated by my distinct lack of enthusiasm for, or desire to engage with, your sense of outrage and injustice.

Picking up your mug, you soften a little and tell me that it makes you so angry. "Me? Or that random story your friend told you on the phone?" This makes you laugh and finally you stand down.

It is not a random story. Apparently this person is always doing this! I watch your hands, notice your frown, hear the tone of your voice and notice the cat, who has been calmly grooming herself, look at you and, tail up, leap off the sofa and mince out.

"The cat has picked up on your anger," I say, giggling. You peer past me at her disappearing out the door and then look at me with your eyebrows up, surprise written across your face.

"Yes, she has picked up the energy of your anger and does not want to be around it."

"She doesn't understand what I'm saying!" you retort. "That is so ridiculous. What rubbish, I've never heard anything so silly."

"Do you like how you are feeling right now?" I inquire gently. I do not look at you as I ask. I am touching the teaspoon on the table, watching my fingers in the sunlight on the cold, gray steel.

It appears you do not, but you ask me to explain my question.

"Notice you are frowning, you have thoughts swirling in your head, you are sharp and ready to be upset."

You nod slowly and now fiddle with your own spoon, turning it over and over, sadly, toward your phone. You check yourself and look at me. "I do not like how I feel, but they ..."

"Yes, I know. Someone else has rattled you and what is interesting is that you have let them. On a normal day, a day when I am not here, what would you go on to do? Now that you have been tripped into anger? Perhaps call someone else and tell them about it? Unconsciously eat a box of cookies? Get into an argument with your partner?"

"Maybe ..." you reply and turn away, looking out of the window. I give you time to think about how you would behave and eventually you sigh and come back to me.

"Yes, I would, but I don't understand how you know this. And why have I never noticed?" you ask. "Say more."

"You allowed yourself to be overtaken, today, by something that has nothing at all to do with you. You are upset about a story that you can do nothing about. It is not yours, on any level, yet you have allowed it to completely change how

you feel. And how you feel affects how you think and behave and, from there, delves into the relationships around you—with your cat, your friends, your partner or the child inside.

"In getting upset, you change the hormonal flow in your body. Your brain changes gears, the muscles in your face tense—hence the frown—your throat constricts, which makes your voice higher and stronger, and your heart rate goes up. You have, in essence, told your brain and body that you are in danger and need to be ready to fight—either to defend or attack."

You look up at me, tearing your gaze away from the window, and ask, "What? Just that phone call did all that?"

I nod and ask, "How many times a day do you feel like this?"

You lean back and laugh, throwing your head back. "So many times a day!"

"Join me in this exercise. OK, sit up." I sit up straight, knees wide, spine straight, inviting you to copy my posture, which you do. "Let's change how you feel …

"Stretch your mouth like this, widen your jaw and pull your lips back to show all your teeth, like a huge yawn. Raise your chin and do it again, this time pulling your shoulders back and pushing your belly forward as you take a huge inhale through your nose, then, as you exhale, relax down. Do it one more time, but this time, as you widen your mouth and stretch up, belly forward, shoulders back, stick out your tongue as far as you can and then relax down on the exhale and close your eyes."

I watch you now, sitting still, breathing gently, and you begin to smile. "How wonderful," you say. "I feel calm and my mind is silent."

"Yes. You have changed how you feel. You have taken your internal stress system and told it that you are safe and all is OK. Your hormonal flow has changed. Now your thinking is gentle, your heart rate normal and your muscles of defense and attack relaxed. You are in a place of presence and calm.

"It is yours, this system, all yours, and you are giving others way too much access to trigger it—and you—into stress and overwhelm.

"A wonderful way to think about all this is: if it is not your circus, they are not your monkeys. Let it go."

The stress system is a wonderful thing. It is also a mighty beast. Quite honestly, I am enthralled by how superb it is.

It is easy to imagine that you find this take on what you may perceive to be your nemesis quite surreal, but read on. This is something that is not taught in schools, is not in common parlance, is not a given and, very sadly until you read this book, is not a go-to.

In pregnancy, with the combination of physical changes taking place in the body and the amount of new information and experiences for the mind to consider, it is likely that we will unconsciously hold tension in the mind and body. We can easily feel overemotional when pregnant and, in this, lose perspective on how we may be overreacting. We are going to take a look at how we function internally in the face of this misunderstood and mistreated rogue part of ourselves in order to best understand how to calm it.

I use the word "rogue" deliberately. A rogue is many things: sometimes delinquent, dangerous and enticing, yet risky, known for being without ethics or scruples. A rogue can also be someone we love; we accept that they are wayward and smile, wisely, at quite how errant and naughty they can be when given the chance, but we know when and how to pull them back. We want to get the rogue on our team to help us, not to send us into tunnels of misery, fury and despair. Those of us who are anxious or compulsive are in thrall to this seemingly errant system, to the rogue.

UNCOVERING YOUR INNER ROGUE

The mind has zero interest in you discovering how roguish it actually is, and it will throw all it can at you to prevent this deeper understanding. However, there is a meditation practice that can help you to learn how mean the mind can be. It is to repeat *I am, I am* silently in your mind for five minutes, over and over—just these four words. They translate into: *I am my soul.*

I am, I am can show you how tricky and wily the mind actually is. Try it and watch your mind do anything it can to hook you out, to take you to your to-do list, to wonder what you are doing later, to tell you to check your phone, to wonder whether the milk is off. The practice, the work, is to recognize that you have been pulled out of *I am, I am* into the humdrum of the mind, and to pull yourself back into *I am, I am*. Recognize, also, that in watching your mind do this, you are already distracted from *I am, I am*. It is a powerful practice in itself.

Take a moment and try the exercise below.

Sit comfortably, spine straight, and set a timer for five minutes. Close your eyes and in your mind play with *I am, I am*. The art is to notice where your thoughts have taken you and, from there, to bring the mind back. I think of the mind as a badly behaved monkey, jumping all over the place to try to escape. You are learning to teach the monkey mind to sit still.

When the timer goes off, sit and reflect for a couple of minutes on what you found your mind did, where it went. This will help you to see quite how naughty it can be.

When I teach about the stress system and how it works, I often tell this apocryphal and idealized story …

Let us imagine that your parents both came together deep in love. Behind them, in their respective stories, there was no trauma or abuse, they were not bullied and they did not have to flee their homelands. Each of their respective childhoods followed this ideal. When you were born, and in your first few months, your mother held, cradled and rocked you, looking lovingly into your eyes as she fed you. Imagine you are watching this play out in a garden in the sunshine. Daddy is standing behind her; his hand rests gently on her shoulder and he is smiling, looking down at the pair of you, and asking Mommy if she needs anything. She smiles at you, feeding you, and then looks up at him with love and says, "No, thank you, all is good." He leaves her with a reassuring squeeze to her shoulder, and her gaze returns to you.

If you could put your little hand down to the grass, you might find a baby deer sitting at her feet and touch its soft head. Birds are singing in the trees above, butterflies flutter lazily around and everything is bucolic, perfect.

Suddenly there is a loud bang and you, the feeding baby, stop and look quickly up at Mommy to see what her reaction is. Funny, babies are so young when they learn to do that. Mommy smiles and calmly says, "Don't worry darling, it's just Daddy shutting the car door."

You know from the tone of her voice and the gentleness of her steadfast and smiling gaze that all is well in your world, and you can greedily return to filling your belly and then, in blissful satiation, doze off. She leans back with you in her arms and closes her eyes to relax while you dream. The baby deer puts its head on its little legs and sleeps, too.

The mother in this story was present, gentle, calm and attuned to you, in her gaze and in her presence. When the loud noise happened, she noticed it, understood what it was and, attuned to your sudden awareness of something you did not understand, she calmed you. You recognized her reassurance and went happily back to feeding. This is attunement.

This is a story that all of us would like, somewhere in our psyche, to have been our own. The personal story of your attunement history forms part of why you are as you are. Maybe for you a version of this story did happen. You may be inherently calm, relaxed and take the world in your stride. Or not. Maybe you are shouty, quick to argue, judgmental or endlessly trying to work out how to soothe and please others.

You may believe that you are genetically like your parents, not only in physical appearance but also in behaviors. You might think that because they were stressed or anxious, this is a permit for you to repeat the cycle. If you are of an anxious disposition, it is easy to think that you will always be like this—fretting, planning, trying to make order out of seeming chaos when no one behaves as you feel they should.

If your growing-up experience was not perfect, then you may begin to understand that you are living in what I call a *pain of the past and fear of the future* mind–body system. This means that you use your perceptions of the past as the lens through which you project and perceive the dramas that may evolve in the present. The brain is endlessly trying to work out how to be safe and, in doing so, it is unaware of the right here, right now. For some, it is challenging to be in the present moment at all. Your *pain of the past and fear of the future* thinking may have been triggered solely by pregnancy. All manner of human experiences can and will put the mind–body axis into a hyperaroused state, where your fight-or-flight response—the sympathetic system—is perpetually "on."

THE SYMPATHETIC SYSTEM

The sympathetic system sounds so lovely and so kind, but trust me, you know when you are in the sympathetic system because it is a terror.

When your mind and body are hyperaroused, taut and contracted, ready to flee or fight, scanning with eyes, nose and ears for the slightest change, you have moved into the more animalistic, survival-based part of your brain: the sympathetic system. Many of us, as a result of experience, spend a lot of time unconsciously moving through our days with an activated stress system. If you have ever watched a fox constantly moving its ears while it feeds on scraps, lifting its head to sniff, eyes roving, then you have seen this system in action.

This branch of us is the part we fly into in a flash, a nanosecond, when we are triggered.

Think about smelling burned toast. You have picked up, through your nose, the smell of smoke. You are compelled to take action, to dash over and throw the offending charred and smoking slice into the sink and open the window.

Or think about those messages pinging on your phone—such a seemingly benign and simple thing that we all take for granted, but notice how they quickly take your gaze and create an imperative to act, to check, to look. Who knows what you will read and where it will take you?

Or think about when you are drifting off to sleep and you notice you haven't felt the baby move for a while. Your system instantly responds with a palpable flush of adrenaline. If you're dozing, your eyes will fly open, you will take a sharp intake of breath, you will raise your head so both ears are uncovered and your eyes may dart around the room as you try to make your thoughts focus. When did you last feel them? If a kick comes, you'll exhale and lie back down …

Your sympathetic stress system has launched itself, full pelt, into your brain, your thinking processes and your body. Once there, unless you are quick to notice it, the sympathetic system, the rogue who can be let loose oh so quickly, will whirl and spin your mind and specific elements of your body into the *pain of the past and fear of the future*. If you are not paying attention, you can become lost in anxious thinking.

This is not a failure on your part, at all; it is just how the stress system works. These are survival instincts and they are paramount. But if you have a tall dark history—perhaps you have experienced previous loss in pregnancy or there is a threat hanging over you—the sympathetic system really does become a monster. For some, it is switched on 24/7. This is the anxious, compulsive, addictive, rageful, fawning and attacking aspect of ourselves.

Because you are pregnant your brain is more attuned to perceived or imagined threats. To be in this state of brain, mind and body all the time is wearing and exhausting, so stress can be compounded in pregnancy as your body is in a period of intense creativity making a baby. Stress hormones intensify issues such as headaches, constipation, sleeplessness and restless legs syndrome, and stress hormones can cross the placental barrier. The baby in your womb, your partner, your pets and your colleagues can all attune to this system because it is catching. It makes them feel unsafe, under threat, watchful and hypervigilant to real or perceived danger. You can also, in turn, find yourself being unconsciously reactive, responding to someone else's anxious facial and vocal communications.

The sympathetic side of the stress system has been weaponized against you by the wide-ranging technology of the twenty-first century, which gathers data and generates financial gain. All of the above creates a complex soup of overwhelm.

This mindset can take a lot of the pleasure out of being pregnant. The nine months of gestation are a unique time in your life and they do, at times, feel as though they are passing in slow motion, yet in the grand scheme of things they flash past.

This is why we want to do conscious breathwork and stretching, so that we can take ownership of this rogue and wayward beast— but more on this in the next chapter. For now, I'd like you to play a game with me.

Get into a relaxed position, perhaps propped up in bed or sitting on a chair. Have a little stretch to make sure you are comfortable. Leave your phone on. And then wait.

It may be challenging to wait, I know, but if you live in the vicinity of people, dogs, a doorbell, you will not have to wait long. Just relax and let your mind wander.

The game is to notice, in your physical body, what happens when you hear a sound like a bang, a bark, a doorbell, a notification chime or a crying child. You think you hear with your ears, but you will have an instant and visceral response to the sound deep in your body. Your heart rate will speed up, your ears will hyperlisten and perhaps your pelvic floor will tighten.

Did you try? Maybe your phone rang or a message came in. Did you notice what happened? Stay with this practice. It takes time to become aware of the visceral nature of the sympathetic system.

THE FOUR PARTS OF
THE STRESS SYSTEM

The stress system, which you are learning is heightened in pregnancy, is made up of four main parts, at least in terms of what you need to know to better understand its function:

1. The vagus nerve
2. The major muscles
3. The amygdala
4. The hormones of stress

These aspects work together in perfect harmony whenever they are called upon: by your history, thoughts and personal surroundings, by noises or by perceived or real threats.

There is much within these pages that has only been discovered in the last 20 years. Research into post-traumatic stress disorder in soldiers began a rapid growth in understanding of the mind–body axis. When we think a stressful thought or are in a stressful situation, the body instantly responds with the activation of the sympathetic system, an escape or defensive transformation in hormones, muscles, organs and senses. As long as this reactivity is unconscious, it is a habit—at times a life-saving one. Neural plasticity means that this habit can be changed over time. We can rewire our thinking, learn to notice when our sympathetic system has been activated and from there become calmer, more responsive, less reactive.

The stretching and conscious breathwork we will explore in later chapters underpin how we rewire the brain—neural plasticity—to be able to better cope with the experience of gestation and, from there, parenting your child.

In the simplest terms, we now know that we can calm ourselves down and, in doing so, ease the physical and emotional aspects of being with child. This is what you will learn to take ownership of as we work through the rest of the book.

The vagus nerve

This is a long and wandering nerve that is bi-directional; it travels up from the pelvic floor and down from the center of the forehead. In women it travels from the vagina, and in men from the root of the penis, up to the forehead. This is the sympathetic route. The parasympathetic route, which we'll explore in the next chapter, runs from the center of the forehead down to the vagina or penis.

The vagus nerve branches into each and every organ of your body, including the lower, animalistic, survival-based part of the brain. Certain major muscles are also affected by it, including the pelvic floor, cervix, diaphragm and larynx.

Moving on down the vagus nerve, we come to the lungs, heart and diaphragm. This section regulates the breathing and heart rate and compresses the diaphragm when triggered to mobilize. The diaphragm is a large muscle shaped like a curved mushroom-top, tucked in under the base of the ribs, which, until you learn to breathe consciously, works automatically in concert with information triggered by the sympathetic state. The tightening of the diaphragm also tightens up the digestive and reproductive organs so that running away is easier.

In the lower part of this journey we find the viscera—hence the phrase "visceral reactions." The pelvic floor, when tight, joins the diaphragm in containing 27 feet of intestines, the liver, stomach and so on. It is the pelvic floor that, when hypertonic (very tight), is the cause of vaginismus and failure to progress in labor. Research suggests that the vagus nerve, in the sympathetic state, controls a wide range of medical issues, including some types of sexual dysfunction, delayed labor, irritable bowel syndrome, constipation, certain digestive disorders, heart attacks, migraines and much more.

When the sympathetic system is mobilized, this nerve contracts all the way through the body to facilitate fight or flight. In the face and throat it is a glorious indicator of danger. The throat constricts so we can shout, scream, speak fast and raise our voice to communicate alarm. The forehead moves in ways that show anger, fear and suspicion, our ears become more alert to sound, our eyes scan and search, and our nostrils flare.

Breathing consciously takes over and softens the vagus nerve.

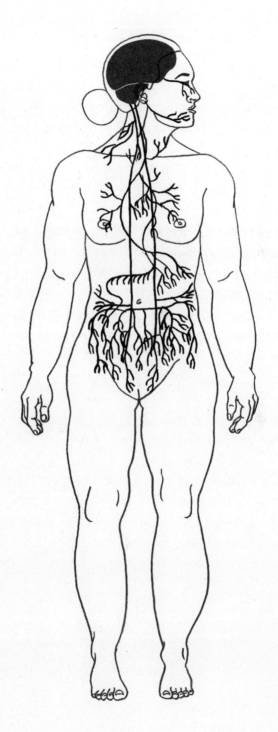

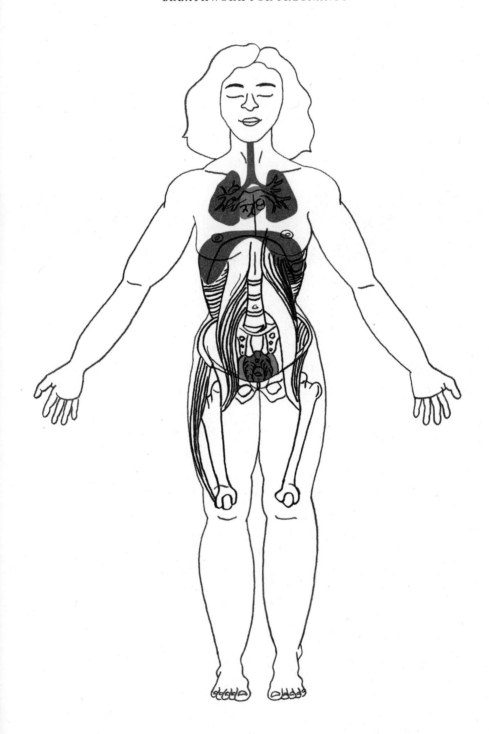

The major muscles

When a trigger mobilizes the sympathetic system, the major muscles contract to aid in any physical reaction that might be needed.

The leg and pelvic muscles

Working our way up the body, we have the thighs; these are the largest muscles in the body, unless you are at full-term pregnancy, in which case the uterus is the largest muscle. Thigh muscles are for running, jumping, resisting and dropping down. They hold an enormous amount of blood when active, hence the sympathetic response compresses the organs above, to push blood down for them to use in escape or defend modes.

The second largest muscles are the psoas. These are made up of three different muscles that wrap around the pelvic bowl and descend to hold your legs onto your torso. It is these three-part muscles that allow you to raise and lower your legs, to walk, run and leap. They are also emotionally linked to our sense of responsibility, and thus backache can be a response to the burden we feel we carry. In pregnancy these muscles come under strain due to the growing uterus. We unconsciously adjust our posture to accommodate and counterbalance—often to our detriment—the forward-carrying weight in later gestation. This strains the stomach muscles and adds more pressure to the lower back. In Chapter 4 there is a story with a magical trick to ease the back, psoas and stomach muscles (see page 81).

In labor the baby travels down through the psoas muscles in the pelvis. These muscles line the back interior of the pelvic girdle and soften the baby's glide out into the world.

The pelvic floor is a thick muscle that holds all the organs below the diaphragm within the body. In a female, the pelvic floor has three openings: the urethra for peeing; the vagina for pregnancy, vaginal sexual intercourse and menstruation; and the anus for bowel movements. It has a range of movement between 4 and 6 inches up and down.

If we have an anxious disposition—for example, if our tall dark history included negative sexual experiences—then we can have a hypertonic (too tight) pelvic floor. This, in turn, is an almost constant trigger to the sympathetic stress system. Learning how to relax the pelvic floor will facilitate a good birth experience.

The adductors lie between the inner thighs and stretch down to the inner knees. They are important to get to know, as they are a part of the folding mechanism that lets you drop down or hide under a table to escape. If the pelvic floor is tight, these may be, too.

In Chapter 4 I will show you how to relax the pelvic floor and the adductors. If this rings alarm bells, please know that the pelvic floor does not hold your baby inside you. The cervix has this role and it manages it superbly. Stretching the pelvic floor will not stretch the cervix. They are independent of each other until the second stage of labor, when they are connected by the child descending from one to the other.

The intercostal and thoracic muscles

Important for breathwork, these are some of the major muscles of respiration and they are impacted by pregnancy in a number of ways.

In stress, they contract, causing the breath to become shallow. In pregnancy, they tend to be stretched out by hormonal changes, but related changes to the ribs mean this isn't always pleasant and welcome.

In pregnancy, the hormone relaxin can cause the intercostal muscles to become softer and stretchier. As a result, the bones in the ribcage often move more than they normally do, and this can cause discomfort. If you have such discomfort, flexing movements backward and forward or on all fours, like "Cat-Cow" (page 104), can help to ease it.

The thoracic muscles, also important for breathwork, are muscles many women become aware of during pregnancy because, to counteract the change to the center of gravity, the thoracic spine is put under more pressure and stress to keep an upright posture. This increases tension through the thoracic muscles and, again, can cause rib and upper back pain.

Stretching before breathwork will help to manage the changes to these muscles and the experience of breathwork.

We now rise up to the larynx, eyes, ears and forehead. These are not large muscles, I know, but they are extremely important relative to the vagus nerve, as they facilitate our ability to communicate surprise, fear and anger. From the throat up to the top of the forehead is the signaling aspect of the vagus nerve. We use vocal tone and facial expressions such as shock, disgust, alarm and anger to communicate with those around us, consciously or not. Working with the stretches and the breaths will soothe facial communication; once you are fully engaged in regular calming practices, you will notice how these signaling aspects of the self are softened over time.

The amygdala

The amygdala is a part of your inner workings and is essential to your relationship with stress on a primal and instinctive level. The amygdala is the part of the brain that keeps us safe. It scans for signs of danger and, in pregnancy, it is heightened to keep the baby safe in your body. Research done on the maternal brain shows that, during pregnancy and the postnatal period, women have increased activity in the amygdala, which, consensus suggests, is an evolutionary move to ensure the mother is fine-tuned to meet baby's needs and keep them safe.

The amygdala sits at the core of our processing of threat, fear and reactivity, in the lower part of our brain. This part of the brain is where we process our basic needs for food, safety, shelter, survival and memory, particularly relative to scary and dangerous experiences, past and current. It is the part of our brain that has allowed us to survive as a species.

The amygdala is made up of two small cashew-shaped glands, one on either side of the brain, and it could be described as the core of the stress system. It is also our amygdala that drives us to tunnel into anxious and projecting thoughts. It processes threatening and fearful stimuli, including looking for and thinking about how to find safety.

This function has also been found, by sheer dastardly chance, to be a major flaw in our brains that now leaves us utterly vulnerable to the more unpleasant aspects of social media, the entertainment industry, mobile phones and the news. It is our amygdala that these industries have learned to infiltrate, attack and weaponize against us.

If we are struggling with a tall dark history, alongside the war being waged upon us by phones and social media (completely by our own free will, may I gently point out), then we are super vulnerable to being triggered. When this happens, we will attempt to ease our unbearable emotional overload—for some this will be through addiction, self-harm or eating disorders; for others it may be through risk-taking behaviors, gambling, raging or obsessive and compulsive disorders.

In the face of smartphones, instant messaging, social media, etc., our little amygdala stands no chance. It is bombarded with relentless threats. In the face of pandemics, climate change, war, flood, famine, heatwaves and fires, what is it to do but stand tall and cry "Help!" *Keep checking, keep scanning, keep liking, keep watching, keep scrolling, keep swiping!* The amygdala will then continue to scan and look for danger, not only on the phone but also in tunnel thinking and wildly projecting into negative future scenarios. When you are also pregnant, your sympathetic stress system can be easily ramped up to intolerable levels, which feels, physically, like a state of complete overwhelm.

In psychotherapeutic terms this aspect of the amygdala is called "negativity bias." To view the negativity bias through the lens of a tall dark history, before computers and smartphones, it was something like 250/1—250 times more biased to the negative than the positive, to look for the negative, to keep scrolling, keep thinking stressful thoughts in an attempt to find safety. This is the protective aspect of the amygdala. Adverse childhood experiences (ACEs) are known to change how the brain is wired and to significantly raise this bias toward seeking safety by being activated into the stress system. Bring in smartphones, combined with the Covid years and all that has been discovered about this flaw in our brains, and we take another mighty leap in our negativity bias up to between 500 and 750/1. The tech companies that run the news, social media and data gathering have weaponized this specific aspect of our humanity and our brains. This means that, for some, negative thinking is the norm and is further reinforced by our use of media and technology.

We have allowed our brains to be 500–750 times more negative than positive. This is hard to read, and it is also hard to live with. Learning how to attune is how you begin to change this bias and rewire your brain.

Because of screens and smartphones, we have so much access to random and unnecessary information. Combine this with personal attendant stress levels, and many people now breathe on average 15 times a minute in their waking lives. That is a shockingly high figure to a trauma therapist, and it is a measure of how much the body and brain are in concert, working together to try to seek out safety. Our stress systems are activated and our brains and bodies are mobilized for escape.

We are all battling with information overload, including triggering posts on social media about loss, birth trauma and negative narratives. The news tells us horror stories about maternity wards and midwives. Data gathering works better when we are triggered and anxious. The purveyors of screens, smartphones, social media and the news have invested a lot of time and money into research-ing how to get us as anxious as possible, as quickly as possible—and you now know this is linked to the amygdala and negativity bias, which are both heightened by pregnancy. It is a well-known fact that when triggered into anxiety we need to search for information, a sense of safety and distraction. Oddly, it seems that we love to be stressed and scared if we feel safe in our homes, hence the rise in violent TV and movies. And if, in our scrolling, we are triggered, we are highly likely to go back and look again, creating a perfect loop, a storm of relentless data capture!

Because of the way algorithms work, if we choose to look at negative stories about birth on social media, we will see more of them. Knowledge can empower, of course, but if you're constantly googling, checking, measuring and testing, then your amygdala is being programmed to look for danger when there is none. At a time when we have been hardwired to be more aware of threats in our surroundings, it is a good idea to practice awareness of how your amygdala is behaving. The choice to sit and breathe will begin to train your amygdala, along with all aspects of the stress system, that it can, if only for a few minutes, stand down.

Your amygdala has been hacked, but with the stretching and breathing tools in this book, you'll learn to hack it back over to your side.

The hormones of stress

In the realm of new discoveries about how our stress system works, hormones play a major role. There are literally thousands of hormonal interactions happening within us all the time, so for our purposes we are going to take a simplified view.

The amygdala, described above, orchestrates the flood of stress hormones in the brain and body. When stressed, our whole hormonal being is transformed, and as pregnancy is a primal state of being, you become more aware of possible threats to you and your baby's safety. It is for this reason that I include this information here.

Adrenaline

You have probably already noticed the presence of adrenaline because you played with the visceral nature of obtrusive noise in the exercise on page 29. Any sound, sight or thought that creates a sense of alarm will deliver a sharp dose of adrenaline into your bloodstream and brain, creating hyperalert noticing. Perhaps you have slept through your alarm and you have a midwife appointment—it is adrenaline that will get you up, dressed and out on time. Adrenaline speeds up the heart and breathing, and in this way channels more blood to the thighs.

Testosterone

Most of us know testosterone as the hormone that drives maleness, fueling young men into fighting and aggression. However, both sexes have testosterone, and its job—other than defining men's deep voices, faster digestion and greater muscle mass—is to support arousal, be it sexual, creative or arousal of anger, rage and fury. When the sympathetic system is triggered, an added burst of testosterone fuels our actions, retorts and attacks. Some women, when carrying a male child, report high levels of sexual arousal, an engorged clitoris and a craving to orgasm frequently. If this is your experience, enjoy! It is normal.

Cortisol

Released when the sympathetic system is activated, cortisol is the most pernicious of the hormones discussed here. If adrenaline is linked to fear activation, cortisol has a more emotional effect. It makes us think stressfully, and so we can use it as a driver to finish an assignment or to get packed and go off on a vacation. However, if cortisol is coursing through your system most or all of the time, then please be aware that it is implicated in almost all illnesses. High levels of cortisol truly disrupt your system in every way. This hormone creates a sense of agitation and endless checking for safety—for instance, looking at the news—perhaps overwhelming those around us with our need for them to make things right or do things to make us feel better, and contributes to the feeling that there is no time, no space, relentless pressure, too much to do. It is the hormone of overwhelm and reactivity.

All three of these hormones can cross the placental barrier, and your child experiences them in terms of elevated heart rate and tension in the vagal system, which is why it is so important to learn how to calm the stress system.

Endorphins

When we are in the sympathetic system, we are generally totally unaware of the sensation or effects of endorphins. Perhaps pre-pregnancy you were a runner. Imagine you've just come back from a great run on a machine or outside; you hit your goal. You have a quick shower, maybe a coffee and charge on with your day, perhaps diving headlong into your phone or going shopping. Either way, you've missed the gift of endorphins because your habits have stopped you from sitting down, being still and really getting into your thoughts: *Wow, that made me feel amazing, so expansive.*

We can also release endorphins by having an orgasm, which really relaxes us, and the afterglow is softening and dreamy.

As we'll explore in the next chapter, this hormone, when you can be calm and still after its release, literally eats up the stress hormones in your body.

In the breathwork chapter, you will learn how to use endorphins to your advantage in preparing for labor.

Dopamine

Now here's a tale to be told. Dopamine is instantly released into the mouth in response to salt, fat and sugar. This is the hormone that has fueled the snack industry and the rise in obesity over the last two decades.

Delving deeper into the story, dopamine has been utterly taken over by our phones. Yes, they, the data and media companies, know, absolutely, that we long for dopamine as it makes us feel connected. Social media, instant messaging, likes and swipes are all built upon the release of a minuscule and totally unfulfilling dose of dopamine. Unfulfilling because it is just not enough to satisfy us, and that sense of lack and wanting more fuels the repetition, the drive to go back in and try again, unsuccessfully, to be satiated. Trust me, if the satisfaction was there the media and tech companies would all be out of business.

We can see how the drive for dopamine is used to seduce us into constantly abandoning ourselves *out there*. When we are in the sympathetic system, our gaze turns away from presence, nature, family and loved ones—you can see this on all forms of transport and in cafes, restaurants, living rooms and bedrooms the world over. Our gaze is tunneled into somewhere else, generally outside of ourselves, or into stressful thinking and the endless need to feel full.

If you are feeling stressed and can relate to this, you can begin to recognize that there is no time to simply be with baby, connected, calm, gentle and present, when you are stressed; it simply does not make sense to be still because the brain and body are mobilized. Imagine how lovely it would be to sit and quietly breathe, eyes closed, after going for a scan and hearing all is well, rather than immediately posting the scan photo on social media and refreshing the screen again and again to read people's responses. Consciously stretching or breathing for a few minutes will make everything calm again.

As you'll learn in the next chapter, when you choose to consciously breathe and stretch, you soothe the vagus nerve, hack the amygdala and change over from hormones of stress to hormones that will better support you.

THE DRAMA CYCLE

When your system is on high alert, consciously or not, you experience the mind and body in a state of protect, attack the other, defend yourself or soothe your assailant, which I call *the drama cycle*.

These behaviors sit in three specific camps: *victim, persecutor* and *rescuer.* They are none of them lovely words, I know.

We will start with the *victim* as the starting point in the cycle, just because somewhere has to be chosen. The first step in the victim role is resentment, and from there you feel as though you are a victim to the other and their behavior. Perhaps they have not asked how your morning sickness has been today or they have not offered to make supper when you are tired and really want to sit still. This can lead to passive-aggressive jibes, stony silence or walking out and slamming the door. Or perhaps your skill is in sulking. Think about how deeply personal and internal pregnancy is for you. You are growing a child—it is *your* mind and body that are so transformed at this time. It can sometimes be easy to have resentful thoughts and feelings.

In this role we can also get angry. Resentments are internalized anger, and some of us like to express these feelings verbally and physically, blaming, trying to control and shaming others. These are only some of the ways that we express our sense of being a victim of the other.

The problem is that, in these expressions of our feelings and our resulting reactive behaviors, we are in fact persecuting the other. Thus we inelegantly move ourselves over to being the *persecutor*, making the other the victim.

We, unconsciously and rather niftily, have got the cycle started and we can keep it rolling for a while—perhaps by constantly switching between the victim and persecutor roles, keeping the fire fueled, so to speak, and throwing the argument back and forth.

Or we might maintain a stony and abandoning silence. We may face away from the other, arms crossed, ablaze with righteous indignation or resentful and poisonous thoughts.

To and fro, back and forth, someone eventually caves and, if their caving is accepted—perhaps with a "sorry" or a kiss, a freshly baked cake or tidying up; you know what you do—just like that, whoever took that brave step is now the *rescuer*, the other is the victim and space is cleared for the whole thing to begin again.

Do my words make sense to you? Can you see that you cycle through these three positions, over and over, on an unstoppable wheel of unhappy feelings, thoughts and behaviors? Can you be aware that learning to attune is a good thing? Would you like agency?

The behavioral description above is the result of an inability to attune, a lack of agency and vulnerable boundaries. It is very common, playing out in most relationships. If you are unconsciously lost to the sympathetic stress response, you are not aware of the process as much as you could be. Your baby is attuned to your state of being and, while none of us can ever get it perfectly right, having a practice of knowing how much impact you can have, as a parent, on how safe your child feels is a lovely thing to begin before they have even arrived.

Because you are pregnant, you are more aware of your surroundings, noises and intrusions into your peace of mind and body. Over the next chapters, we will explore how we can use breathwork and stretching to find a way through this endless muddle of hurt and abandonment. We will be together as you learn how to land in gentle, calm presence and, from there, to know when and how to change how you feel.

MENTAL HEALTH ISSUES

Mental health issues abound in this stressed world. It is unlikely that many, if any, of us will escape without some experience of them in our lives. I include anxiety, depression, a history of ACEs, obsessive-compulsive disorder and addictions in the term "mental health."

There is a spectrum of issues we could cover here, but for each sufferer of any of those mentioned above, it can all be defined as suffering.

For some, anxiety is chronic (i.e., long term), while some is situational (meaning the extremes of the current moment in time). Anxiety can be alleviated by stretching and breathwork; this is an accepted medical fact. For example, taking an overview of yoga audiences, a large percentage do yoga for the alleviation of stress, anxiety and mental health recovery. All of the stretches and breaths in Chapters 4 and 5 will positively impact your state of mind and being. You could take a moment now and try the "Arm, Chest and Back Stretches" (page 106) followed by "Single Nostril Breathing" (page 129).

Low-grade depression is eased by movement, stretching and breathwork. The "Alternate Arm and Leg Raises" (page 114) stimulate and energize the body. Combine this with "A Breath to Manage the Mind" (page 134) and you will have changed how you feel and think.

Some issues, such as severe depression, do require mental health experts. If you were on medication pre-pregnancy and have now come off it, do keep an eye on your mood and revisit your doctor or mental health service to discuss your needs.

Chapter 2

The Power of the Breath

We are busy. Pregnant or not, the garden awaits. Sitting on the ground weeding a flower bed in the sunshine, I can see that you are finding the process dull. You get angry with weeds that are reluctant to be pulled. Your knees hurt, as you have already said several times, and you are still smarting from an earlier argument with your partner.

Forehead crinkled in a frown, you huff and puff. Eventually you sit back and give up, throwing aside the latest tuft of vegetation, arms folded, pouting like a petulant child.

I sit back with you and invite you to stretch out your legs. You sigh and do as I ask.

"This is a perfect time and place to show you something," I say. Your reply is grumpy; it is clear you are not in the mood.

I lean back and look up at the blue sky with a smile. This is as irksome, my smiling, as the weeding, you say, and you go on to tell me that I don't know what it is like to be you.

"Tell me how you feel."

"Pissed off and misunderstood" is the churlish reply.

"OK." I nod. "This is a perfect feeling. It makes sense of how you are being, and it is a feeling that can easily be cultivated into resentment or a fight for later."

You cast me a sideways glance. I obviously do understand.

"How does your face feel? The muscles in your face?" I ask, watching your jaw clenching and the deep furrow between your eyebrows.

"*Tight, stressed*" *is your answer, which I feel shows good self-awareness—and it is obvious, too.*

"*What about your inner self? Where do you feel it?*"

Your answer is perfect: in your head, which is relentlessly playing over the morning's events, and in your chest, which is tight, the angry kind of tight. Yes, I know it well, that feeling.

"*Do you want to stay like this?*" *I gently ask, picking a small daisy and twirling it in my fingers.* "*Or do you want to change how you feel?*" *I turn and offer you the daisy.*

This makes you throw your head back and laugh. "*Ha! How on earth can I change how I feel? Once you feel something, you're stuck with it!*" *you reply.*

I am undaunted; we are now exploring the perfect mood for me to show you how easily and effectively you can transform your emotional and physical self.

"*Play a game with me,*" *I implore.* "*Will you try something?*"

You nod with little charm, sigh and sit up.

"*Can you cross your legs again, or do you prefer to sit as you are, wide-legged?*" *You pull your feet in and sit in what is called "easy pose," cross-legged.* "*Perfect.*" *I smile and pull myself around to sit in front of you on the blanket.*

"*How you are thinking and how you are feeling are in perfect concert. I know it feels awful to you, and I am not making fun of you. You have a system activated in your body, a system we all have, which doesn't come with a user's manual. You have never been shown how to manage this unruly internal mechanism.*"

This makes you smile, sit up a little straighter and wriggle your shoulders to get more comfortable.

"*Just do as I do, copy me for a few breaths, and then let's check in with how you are feeling. Is your belly comfortable? Do you need a pillow to raise you up a little?*"

"*Yes.*" *You take it and put it under your pelvis, straightening your posture.*

"*Sit beautifully.*" *This makes you giggle as you look down at yourself, covered in mud.* "*Put your hands on your knees and keep your spine straight.*"

We are going to do a simple, five-second breath.

"*You are going to inhale through tight lips for about five seconds, hold for a moment, then exhale through your nose for five seconds. Let's try one round and go from there. Copy me."*

I tighten my lips and there is a gentle hissing sound as I take five seconds to inhale through my mouth. "Hold for a moment. Now a gentle exhale through your nose." You nod. "Close your eyes and let's do ten rounds together.

"Let the breath go as deeply into your stomach as you can. Don't hold it up in your ribs; relax the belly and lift the torso up as you inhale, gently softening the torso down on the out-breath. Try to keep your face soft, no frowning."

You are doing well and also, I note, remembering to hold for a moment at the top of the in-breath. Your eyes sneak a peek at me and I gently remind you to close them.

This is the last two rounds. "At the end, stay still, just breathe gently, eyes closed. I will not move or leave. Can you sit for a minute or more?"

After the time has passed I ask, "What are you thinking?"

You open your eyes and look straight at me. "I am not thinking about anything! How can that happen? How did my mind stop?"

"And feeling? How are those tight and angry feelings?"

"They have gone."

Everything is quiet and slow and the baby is moving in your belly; the sensation of quickening makes you put your hand down to the movement and smile. You feel gentle and calm, you say, looking up, now, in wonder at how blue the sky looks.

"OK," you say. "Tell me what you just did to me!"

I laugh and say it was not me. It was you. You changed how you felt, you breathed consciously and slowly, as this breath asked, and the result is that you have changed both your mind and your emotional body.

I stand up and offer you my hand to help you rise gently to standing.

Come with me, keep reading and I will explain.

It is an option to career at high speed through this life, oblivious, stressed, overwhelmed, blind to the present moment and all your innate possibilities, wallpapering everywhere around you with your story. You can numb yourself with swiping and liking, arguing and living in an endless cycle of triggers, always on the lookout for the next drama. You can find yourself becoming bogged down with the discomforts of pregnancy, such as morning sickness, tiredness, backache or constipation, believing that there isn't another way.

But there *is* another way. You can choose—taking in and using all that I gift you here—to be present. Present to the here and now, to your growing baby, to your part in the world and its magic, opening continuously, you as a microcosm of the cosmos, endlessly expanding. Pregnancy is a time you will always remember. To pause, soften, be still, be present allows you to really cherish this time and form long-lasting memories and stories to share with your child.

In the previous chapter we explored what it looks like when your sympathetic system is activated. Now I want to show you that you can learn how to take over this system and, in doing so, own your stress system for yourself. You can decide when you want to calm down, become still, be present.

This means that you can change how you feel. It is an amazing thing anyone can do and yet for some wild and crazy reason it is the biggest secret in the world! And what is even more wonderful in learning this wild and crazy secret is that, as you change how you feel, your baby will change with you!

When you are stressed, the child inside or outside you is stressed, too. So is your cat, your dog, your partner—everyone around you is affected by this state; they share and respond to your stress hormones. Choose to calm yourself down and peace will return to your world, both internal and external.

We meet in this chapter so that I can explain how, through breathwork, stretches and sitting in gentle silence after either or both, you will discover that you have the agency to change how you think and feel. Agency means you are in charge of your responses.

Perhaps you are easily triggered, judgmental, angry, resentful or overly helpful, or perhaps you have a tendency to make cutting remarks to hurt and push others away. In all of these behaviors you do not have agency. You are at the mercy of the safety mechanisms that run through your mind and body. For some, particularly those with an anxious or irascible disposition, this can be happening all the time. Others may experience it only with certain people or in particular situations. For most of us our reactivity is a default position, meaning we jump into it, unthinking, and this unconscious reactivity can be easily heightened in pregnancy.

Your mind and body belong to you, not to the whims and vagaries of the other. Awoken to your agency, you can notice that a look or a situation makes you feel uncomfortable. From there, rather than rushing into instant and perhaps repetitive reactivity, you can take a moment, reflect on how what happened has rippled through your mind and body, and consider your position in terms of how to behave and think.

You will learn, in these pages, that agency means you can adjust yourself to the situation; you can choose to take a moment and consider whether you need to be upset, anxious or reactive. Can you allow yourself to recognize that, in pregnancy, you are more likely to be more alert to all that is happening around you, and take a moment to reset? Would a stretch and a breath technique be useful now?

This is not to say that there will not be unexpected events, emergencies and realities. But even in these times the breath can allow you to have mastery over yourself—to slow down your own internal panic, to take agency.

During pregnancy and post-birth it is empowering to recognize this agency. However your pregnancy is playing out, having periods of quiet reflection—times at which you can regroup, take time for you, allow your brain to decompress—will mean you sleep better, feel more positive about the future and are better able to connect to your baby.

As you move toward becoming a parent (and I respect that you may already be one), you are given the exquisite opportunity to change how you behave relative to how you think and feel—all through the power of the breath.

THE PARASYMPATHETIC SYSTEM

The parasympathetic system is another state of the mind and body, the flipside to the sympathetic system, which we can access through stretching and conscious breathing. We can take over the sympathetic system that we explored in the last chapter and move over—brain, mind and body—to the parasympathetic system. I like to think of it as sending in the paramedics to provide instant assistance, relief, utter transformation.

The landscape of the parasympathetic system is open-hearted, gentle, calm, accepting and allowing. There is time, there is space. In this, there is no urgency, no drive to survive at all costs. The heart rate slows down, the amygdala settles, the hormonal flow changes and major muscles in the body relax as you take yourself out of reactivity. You respond, notice, reflect. This is agency.

Our organs, including the nose, ears and eyes, can smell the roses, listen to the birds and be here—right here, right now—for ourselves and others. You will be ready, if triggered, to mobilize again, but over time you will be less and less taken by the mighty beast, the rogue that is the sympathetic system. You will learn to respond, attune and be present. You will find calm in your pregnancy journey.

It is easy to turn to a breath description in Chapter 5 and try it out, having no idea why it works and how it changes you. Sit, set a timer and have a go. Why not? But should you wish to go deeper, by reading this chapter to understand what you are doing and what it is *doing to you*, you will find the experience of breathing and stretching very different. This knowledge gives you agency.

THE FOUR SECTIONS OF THE PARASYMPATHETIC SYSTEM

As you know by now, I am not lots of things—not a doctor, not a physiotherapist, not a brain scientist. However, in this section, the goal is once again for you to get an understanding of how and why breathwork and stretching have such an impact on both your physical and mental states.

Let's start by looking at the main aspects of the parasympathetic system:

1. The vagus nerve
2. The diaphragm
3. The hormones of presence
4. The spinal nervous system

The vagus nerve

In the last chapter, our gaze was on how the vagus nerve is activated through the sympathetic system. Making friends with your vagus nerve is a great way to improve your mental, emotional and physical health. Breathwork is, in my experience, the most accessible, simplest and loveliest way to do this. Calming the vagus nerve can also be done in a huge number of other ways, including stretching.

You consciously move over to the parasympathetic system when you stretch the hips and pelvic floor, the diaphragm, chest, ribs, armpits, throat, mouth and tongue, and relax tension in the face, jaw and lips. In choosing to stretch, to breathe, you release the contraction of the internal organs and major muscles.

The vagus nerve is in the lips, too, and smiling can help to release the tension you feel, especially when you smile with your eyes. The vagus nerve responds to the change, for the better, in your facial muscles.

Let's get to know the sensation of calming the system. Read through the exercise below first so you understand what you are doing. Your eyes will be closed as you play with this process. Each step asks for three gentle breaths.

This exercise is called the Inner Smile.

Sit comfortably tall with the spine straight and set a five-minute timer when you are ready to begin.

Starting with your face, imagine that your eyes and mouth want to smile. Let this happen—actually smile and feel how that makes your eyes soften.

Your ears want to relax and smile. Take your attention to them and soften the muscles around them.

Now your throat wants to soften and smile. Notice how this opens the larynx, the muscles of the throat.

Your shoulders are next to want to join in. They will soften and lower as they smile.

It is the ribcage that longs to smile now. Take a deep breath into the ribs as they smile and open wider and the lung capacity deepens.

Moving down, the diaphragm (the large muscle under the ribs) is ready to smile, and as you take the next inhale, allow your belly to relax and expand further than it has in your pregnancy thus far.

The intestines want to smile, too. Imagine the stomach, liver, spleen and all the feet of intestines relaxing into the "rest and digest" state.

In your mind's eye, go into your uterus, to the baby inside, and see them smile and the uterus become soft, comfortable and peaceful in its daily tasks.

Your last smile is into your pelvic floor. It may be the first time you have invited this large muscle to relax and soften into a smile.

Stay in this softened place, breathing gently into your belly. If you notice you are frowning or your jaw is tight, kindly ask for a smile again.

Bask in this space where you have explored the vagus nerve on its route through your body.

The diaphragm

The diaphragm is a smooth muscle, which means it automatically responds and adjusts to signals from the sympathetic and parasympathetic systems. When we breathe consciously, we do a wonderful thing; we totally take over this automatic function and control the breath ourselves.

By working through the stretching and breathing exercises in this book, you will be able, through practice, to hold yourself in the soothed and gentle state for increasing lengths of time. This ability to recognize, stabilize and transform the state of being signals all your organs to get back to their normal functions.

The hormones of presence

Let us now take a look at the hormonal changes that are brought about in the transition over to the parasympathetic system.

When you consciously take control and agency over your stress system, adrenaline, testosterone and cortisol all stand down (reducing stress hormones in pregnancy is important) and your face and vocal tone soften. You are no longer the harbinger of dread and doom, someone to be wary of or triggered by. Instead you are easy to be around, safe to play beside, perhaps even fun to be with. You are attuning to yourself and your baby.

Dopamine

In the parasympathetic state of being, you have access to dopamine just from smiling and stretching, and also because you are no longer feeling or reacting to a sense of threat. You can sit back and relax, perhaps even read a book. Salt, sugar and fat are now no longer needed to soothe you.

Serotonin

Serotonin is a really interesting hormone that is only released in abundance when we are in our parasympathetic system. (When in the sympathetic system only 5 percent of the available serotonin is supplied, as it would be counterintuitive to provide more if stillness is anathema.)

Serotonin is a wonder hormone that has many varied roles, but for our purposes 95 percent of serotonin is released by the proper functioning of your gut and it is an important hormone for your well-being. Low levels of serotonin can be linked to depression. When you move into the parasympathetic system, your gut releases serotonin because the vagus nerve is relaxed, and this in turn releases the contraction of the intestines and they move into digestion rather than mobilization mode. The resulting release of serotonin makes you feel safe—safe enough to be still.

Let us play with the sensation of releasing serotonin.

Stand up with your feet comfortably apart. If balance is an issue, rest a thigh against the sofa or a table for balance. Tuck in your pelvis—this means lifting your pubic bone at the front and thus supporting your lower back. Stretch up on the inhale, taking care not to have too much of a sway in your back, and open your arms wide, then twist round, shoulder and head, to one side with a deep exhale. Inhale back to the center and twist to the other side, again on the exhale. You want to feel the twist in your diaphragm and either side of your bump.

If you're not too far into the pregnancy and can still stand and fold over with your legs comfortably apart, inhale to the center, head low, and exhale around each foot. Slowly come back up, walking your hands up your legs to be kind to your back.

Sit down and take a moment to notice how still your mind and body have become. This is serotonin.

When you move through flexes and twists, as far as is possible and comfortable in pregnancy, you massage and compress the intestines. As a thank-you, they gift you serotonin. It really is as simple as that. Deep, belly-releasing breaths, where the relaxation of the stomach muscles pushes the diaphragm down, also squish the innards, and the body and brain are rewarded anew. It is easy, then, to sit back after a stretching or breathing practice and gather up all that lovely serotonin to further repair the effects of too much stress on your neural plasticity. Serotonin release makes it easy to be present, still and calm.

DHEA

Dehydroepiandrosterone (DHEA), only released in the parasympathetic system, is said to be the opposite to cortisol as it is only released when this stress hormone is at low levels.

In many of the breaths to come, you will notice I use a five-second inhale and the same on the exhale, releasing the belly as I inhale. Studies on the potency of the breath—particularly those that recognize that we have neural plasticity available to us—have found that the five-second breath is a good way to regulate our diaphragm and thus take us into the parasympathetic system.

You are always invited to be still and present after each breath, and it is in this space, breathing slowly below the diaphragm— meaning that only the belly moves, as this large, curved muscle rises and descends—that we release DHEA, when we can take peaceful, slow, five-second-inhale and five-second-exhale breaths through the nose. You have used the breath to take yourself into the parasympathetic system and therefore your cortisol levels have reduced. From here, DHEA is released to generate a feeling of wellness. The post-breathwork stillness takes you to this specific and beneficial hormonal landscape within yourself. You want to bask in this quiet five-seconds-in, five-seconds-out relaxation, to let it wash over you, lapping gently, like the softest waves, through organs and brain, saying, "Thank you, thank you, thank you." This is its job, to create that specific sensation of wellness for you and your baby.

Oxytocin

Oxytocin, released by the pituitary gland, is the hormone that starts natural labor. If you are planning to be induced, the hormone they use to do this is a synthetic form of oxytocin, Pitocin, administered intravenously. While the body's hormonal cascade triggered by natural labor can promote the release of endorphins to help relieve pain, this phenomenon tends not to occur with the introduction of Pitocin.

We release oxytocin in many ways. The amygdala has a high concentration of receptors for oxytocin, and both the number of these receptors and our levels of oxytocin surge during pregnancy. While the amygdala is hypervigilant and scanning for danger, oxytocin helps you to bond, stay focused during feeding times and make sure your baby is safe. Oxytocin allows you to connect.

Oxytocin has been shown to increase when women look at their babies, or hear their cries, or snuggle with them. This means that, although your amygdala will be watching for danger to your baby by looking over and at them, you will also experience brain changes that are similar to the responses and changes that happen to the brain when you are falling in love.

The increase in oxytocin during breastfeeding is thought to explain why breastfeeding mothers are more sensitive to the sound of their babies' cries than non-breastfeeding mothers.

Oxytocin is the hormone of love, of bonding, of connection. It is present when we are really present to, and in love with, our life as it unfolds before our eyes.

Endorphins

We come back around to endorphins, now, as experienced in the parasympathetic system. Here we have a type of endo-morphine, an opiate, released *as the result of effort.*

This does mean that getting your endorphins requires effort and in the effort—particularly in the arm movements in the section on breaths for the build-up to labor (page 191)—you may feel discomfort. You could say, "No, I feel pushed, stressed by this posture. Surely this is not right!" I can see why, given all that we now know, but would you say this if you were going for a run, or to the gym, or getting all hot and sweaty making love? Endorphins are also released by orgasm. You know now that the reward for the effort is this hormone, which not only makes you feel dreamy and expansive, and hence increases your trust that you can and do release it, but also builds up your tolerance of discomfort to support natural labor, if you want it.

Endorphins serve another important purpose. When you are deeply relaxed, after challenging breath and arm work, after great sex or when you are deeply asleep (yes, endorphins are released in deep natural sleep), they have a mighty task: they eat up, gorge on and gobble up all the stress hormones that we met in the previous chapter. It is good practice for your whole internal self to be still and gentle when you know you have made a major physical effort. Trust me here.

The spinal nervous system

The spine is made up of a series of vertebrae, stacked one on top of the other from your sacrum in your pelvis.

Within the vertebrae, the spinal cord rises up into the skull and the brain. The spinal cord never connects to the vagus nerve; these are two separate and differently functioning main nerves. From the spinal cord, all the major nerves branch out into the arms, pelvis and legs, and if you are experiencing the common pregnancy ailment of sciatica (see page 91 for more on this), this is due to the sciatic nerve being pinched in its passage from the spinal nervous system through the sacrum. The spinal cord does not regulate organ function.

Bathing the spinal cord and the brain are approximately 125 milliliters of transparent lumbar cerebrospinal fluid. Each of us make between 600 and 750 milliliters of this liquid a day, and it has its own pulse. It is not known whether it is our heart or our breathing that causes this wave to travel continuously up and down the spinal cord and around the brain, which floats in a sea of this fluid. It is thought to be a part of the lymph system and to carry hormones in the body. It seems likely that this substance also washes the brain when we sleep, going in and clearing up waste from all the thinking, using endorphins released in relaxed sleep to do so.

I bring you the lumbar cerebrospinal fluid pulse wave as an offering, not from me, but as an extraordinary part of your physical being that you can access within yourself after breathwork when in the parasympathetic system. With practice, you will become familiar with a very particular place within yourself where the muscles and organs have relaxed, the hormones have changed over and you are basking in serotonin, dopamine, endorphins and DHEA. You will find that this induced state of presence allows you to rock gently with the pulse of this magical fluid. It is a gentle swaying from the base of the pelvis—subtle but not imperceptible. In all my years of practice and sitting to enjoy the altered state of being in such holistic peace, this pulse is always the gift at the end.

You gave a version of this exercise a try on page 23. Try it again now and see if you can begin to notice how this positive action changes your internal landscape.

Sit up tall and straight, knees wide, roll your shoulders, push your belly forward, stretch your arms up, raise your chin and stick out your tongue. Repeat this action three times and then sit still, gentle and quiet for a moment.

You have done a number of things to your body, all positive and relevant to this section on hormones. Stretching releases dopamine into the system. Hooray! You can give yourself dopamine. If you can sit quietly now, you might notice that there is a rather lovely feeling in your body. The vagus nerve has been stretched and released, the hormones have changed over and the major muscles have lengthened and softened.

You have stretched and landed in the here and now. You are becoming more familiar with the changes you can effect.

USING THE BREATH TO FIND CALM

In the meeting that opened the first chapter, we looked at anger and how it is often used to moderate intimacy and family situations. Beneath the anger, we found fear and a sense of abandonment.

Take a moment to reflect on the five-second breath you tried on page 49 (if you did not try it, go back and do so now). Did you notice that you felt better afterward? That you softened your reaction to being confronted with your own behaviors as you read? It is likely the scenario created a frisson, some anxiety perhaps, in your body and mind. Were you able to take the time and notice that you had softened? That you had brought change to what you thought and felt in response to the imagined scenario?

If you were calm and gentle in response to this, you actually achieved attunement through these actions, and from there, agency. Well done.

In breathwork you have access to an extraordinary gift, and as your practice settles and you become an adept, because of all you are learning here, you will be able to access a state of calm presence that is quite extraordinary.

You will not always, at the start of this endeavor, be able to be calm, to notice. This may be because you are interrupted, or perhaps you are so hyperaware both of sound and other people that it is not safe enough to be calm. Be patient with me and with your-self—this can take a little practice. And as you are here to learn, practicing is important.

Just as we have within us a hair-trigger ability to mobilize and escape, we also have within us the ability to be calm. Let me start by defining "calm." To be calm is to have a quiet mind and gentle breathing. It is body, hormones, muscles and organs all peacefully doing their daily tasks with little or no disturbance. When put to flight, like a flock of scared pigeons, these parts of you, alongside your conscious awareness, can be soothed back down. When you take stock, consider your options and see the bigger picture of what you want, breathwork and stretching will give you the time and space to calm back down to a centered being, living *right here, right now.*

So please, put down your phone.

Sit back for just a moment and reflect upon the possibility of taking on such a curious journey. It is deeply counterintuitive to the turbulent thoughts and feelings that may inhabit your version of reality on a daily basis. The seduction of watching, checking, scanning, scrolling, liking and sharing is a magnetic cloud that exists completely outside of you.

Calm is always available to you, but our brains and emotions have been turned far, far away from finding the path.

To walk toward that unfamiliar experience, if you can allow the journey to unfold, you have to begin by putting down some of the safety mechanisms you have in place.

As an example, you may be reading this with your phone, as ever, in sight. A stream of one-line text messages starts coming in—ping, ping, ping. You *have to* look, you *must* know, even if it's exasperating.

But do you *have to*? Do you *really*? You may now begin to see, to understand that we can cast our gaze to a different horizon. Remembering our earlier meetings, you could turn your phone over, stretch and go back to reading.

Perhaps a conflict somewhere is endlessly diverting your news viewing into tunnels of awfulness. It *is* awful, but can you do anything, on a personal level, to make a difference? Or is it just fuel for fury? You could decide to make a donation and, in that, know that you have done all you feasibly can, and thus step away.

This is taking a position that is more neutral. Neutral does not mean you do not care—it means you can stay calm in the face of it. If you're really agitated, you can change how you feel.

Let me ask you three questions. I hope you will write down your responses on a piece of paper, with a pen, thereby exercising faculties that are little used now in the face of phones. Perhaps you can prop the piece of paper up on a vase of flowers after you have finished, then sit comfortably and reflect. The ability to reflect is part of being calm—it bears no judgment. By contrast, to be reactive demands action, creates an imperative to judge. Sometimes this is needed, but not all the time.

1. Do you deserve to be calm?
2. When do you feel safe?
3. When do you feel unsafe?

These questions ask you to reflect. Write on a separate piece of paper for each one.

Exploring the first question, what comes up for you? Maybe thoughts like these run through your head:

- The baby's room needs painting.
- I have no time to be calm.
- We have not made the crib yet.
- I need to buy baby clothes.

You may notice that, until now, you have found being calm quite tricky; you've never really known how to find it or how to stay calm. And if you are calm, how will all the tasks get finished?

See what comes up for you in this question and perhaps you can connect to more than my suggestions.

The second question can elicit some rapid answers, but you may be surprised that they are also very specific. Suggestions to help you could include:

- when I feel the baby move
- when my partner cooks supper
- when I am with friends
- in bed with the baby safe in my tummy
- in the supermarket
- when my partner comes home at night and shuts the front door

My suggestions may be helpful, but kicking against them and thinking, *No, none of these*, can also help you get in touch with where safety lies for you.

The third question is the one that you will perhaps reflect on for longer than the others:

- when strangers touch my belly without asking
- when other people tell me their birth stories
- standing pregnant on a bus filled with rowdy schoolkids and no one has offered me their seat
- taking the bins outside in the dark, pregnant and lifting the garbage
- when a friend is gossiping about another mother

You may have instant responses to these questions and yet, on reflection, you may also notice more to add to your answers over the coming days.

These three questions are a potent tool that will help you to notice your stress system or, conversely, when you are calm and peaceful. When you notice that you feel safe, tell yourself you feel safe. This will positively reinforce your new awareness and aid neural plasticity.

Particularly in the case of ACEs, a daily reset to the parasympathetic system through breathwork trains the brain, body and emotional self to become resilient. We want, as parents, to find resilience so that we can hold difficult feelings and emotions without falling into the despair of the victim–persecutor–rescuer drama cycle (see page 44).

As we work through this book together, we can alleviate your stress, fear and anxiety—we can choose to slow it all down, calm the mind and make space for you, in your mind and body, where everything can go quiet and you can become present. From this place, you can begin to recognize your agency, recognize that you have a choice to soothe and soften the triggers when they come so that tunneling into negative/anxious thinking becomes a less unconscious behavior.

In this way, you will hold less stress, tightness and tension in your body, your baby will feel calmer (whether or not they are still in utero) and you will model for them that while it is OK to be affected by negative emotions, it is possible to move through them and create change in how you feel, so that those negative emotions don't move into other parts of your day/week/life and have a negative impact on others, too.

We can choose to take ourselves—notice the language here: *choose* to take ourselves—into a new mental and physical landscape, and access more of our brain, too. Our amygdala can be told to stand down. You will learn that you can say to the monster rogue, "Thank you, I am OK, I have got this."

THE BREATH CAN BE A SACRED PRACTICE

When you choose one of the breaths in Chapter 5, this is, in itself, a conscious act of connection with a transformational practice. You are making a decision to do something for yourself—perhaps for sheer pleasure, perhaps to calm your mind-and-body system. You are connected to a deep need, within yourself, to experience a different state.

When you begin to connect, to allow the breath to flow in and out, to work with the timing, you are connecting to stillness, to presence, to the now. Think of it as pulling in the tangled and complex thought processes that are all whirring away, high up above your head. When we are stressed, anxious or unhappy, our mind machinates, makes stories, goes running toward more stress. It is its own, seemingly unstoppable force.

It may not come until the end of a breath, and it may take practice, but you *will* connect to the now. Right here, right now.

Presence facilitates a connection to and with nature—not just our nature, within ourselves, but the sky, the clouds, the rain, the weeds that grow so energetically from a crack in the pavement. You can witness the now. You can appreciate and be with the world on this day, and land into your belly, the growing baby and others around you.

Going one step further in connection, breath manipulation is also known as pranayama in Sanskrit. It is one of the eight limbs of yoga. Alongside posture, meditation and prayer, it is an excellent way to manage stress.

Doing breathwork is to sit with the Divine, to inhale and exhale the Divine. The inhale is to inspire: *inspirare* in Latin, to take in the spirit. To exhale is to expire: *expirare*, the spirit leaves you, in essence, dies. It is a way of consciously playing with the cycle of life and death.

From all that you have read you know that to take over the amygdala and the vagus nerve is to take over the anxious body. Pranayama or conscious breathing is the route to gaining true mastery over the mind.

Chapter 3

The Three Minds

We are going on a walk as I explain this. We meet on a damp, foggy, gray day. The sun is hiding.

"When you discovered you were pregnant, did you decide to be really positive all the way through the process?" I ask you, in the hazy, creeping damp.

You smile and then laugh, turning to look at me as we walk.

"In your daily life do you ever make resolutions, new year or not, to be more positive?"

You smile and nod, looking down as we walk.

"Let's sit here." I point to a long bench and lean my large umbrella against the end of it. "We can watch the ducks emerge and fade with the fog as we talk."

You tell me about saying to your partner and friends that you would be positive all the way through the 40 weeks, and how challenging that is for you. It is a short story about trying to withhold negative thoughts, and you end by laughing gently but looking away. We are both quiet for a while, watching the water lapping at the shoreline.

I turn to you and you look at me.

"It is a wonderful thing, the stress system. It is so very determined that it knows best that it has all the exits covered. Stress, fear, anxiety, overwhelm—they are all part of the same mindset, and in this challenging time, in the vast cycles of time, not just in your body but in the twenty-first century, we can see how our stress and anxiety levels have been hijacked. Can you relate to how the negativity bias affects focus and creates an overwrought need to check all is safe?"

You frown and at the same time nod, lips pursed as you breathe out and seem to soften a little. Yes, it is all coming together.

"Do you remember that you are learning new tools? You are learning to be, to actually become, conscious of this shift and, from there, choose to manage and change how you feel."

"Yes." You sit up. You have stayed with your commitment to use social media only once a day for 20 minutes, even though you can see how seductive it is to keep looking. I smile at you and say, "Great. Well done."

"Through the lens of breathwork there are three states of mind: negative, positive and neutral. Each is a very different state of being and most of us only recognize the polarities of negative and positive." I turn to you as I ask, "Does it make sense, now, to have negative first?"

"It is not how we usually put those words, positive and negative, together," you explain. "So yes, it jars on several levels."

I can understand this. "Who wants to be seen as having a negative mind, especially when pregnant?" I ask. This makes you smile and you lean back, your face tilted up, eyes closed. You know the negative mind very well, it would seem.

"Ha!" you say, quietly. "No one has ever asked me to become conscious of how I think when I am stressed." You nod slowly. "How do you know when you are in the negative mind?" you ask me, face still, eyes closed, a light rain falling now.

I put up the umbrella over us and, leaning back, begin to explain to you what I find quite so entrancing about this wild beast. "The negative mind describes a very particular state of being. Did you hear the word 'being'?"

You nod expectantly.

"Let us dive a little deeper. Get comfortable."

You wriggle; you are in love with the sound of the rain on the taut material over our heads—and listening to me, you quickly reassure me.

THE NEGATIVE MIND

You now know that the stress system utilizes four separate internal systems, all of them intertwined, all reacting or responding, depending on the state of the mind and body, in perfect harmony with each other. When stressed or anxious, brilliantly quickly, blindingly quickly, speed-of-light quickly, you are in the negative mind. There is generally no conscious awareness of the shift, but you can know you are there in two main ways.

The first is rooted in your sensations. Here are some questions to help you notice when you are, in essence, lost in the realms of fear and uncertainty:

- Are you frowning?
- Are your ears tight, hyperlistening, straining to hear sounds your brain will interpret as information? Or are you holding your breath, frozen, ear cocked, straining to hear more? What was that? Are they home? Are they angry?
- Do you need to keep checking social media or the news, to keep touching your phone, scanning for likes?
- Are your lips tight?
- Are you clenching your jaw?
- Is your mouth dry?
- Is your chest or heart area tight?
- Is your breathing fast and shallow?
- Is your foot tapping, your leg jiggling?
- Are you feeling frightened and possibly also tearful?
- Do you feel childlike, small and alone?

These are some of the physical signs that you are in the negative mind.

The second, your thinking, is another great indicator:

- Are you being negative? Thinking that you'll be a terrible mother? Or that you won't get the birth you want? That something's going to go wrong?
- Have you separated yourself out and away from the situation?
- Do you think no one else could possibly understand how hard pregnancy has been for you?
- Do you feel out of place at your prenatal classes? That the others don't like you?
- Are you waiting for the end of the world?
- Are you wildly projecting? Thinking of all the worst-case scenarios for how things may be during or after the birth?
- Are you shaming or berating yourself? Thinking that you shouldn't feel like this? That you're meant to be grateful and happy all the time because you're pregnant?
- Are you thinking of acting out in some way (e.g., shopping for random nothings, gambling, binge-watching violent TV, going out for that large, frosty-cold tub of ice cream)?
- Are you snapping at your partner? Telling them you don't want them at the birth? Snapping at your midwife?

We can be highly judgmental of our negative mind, and we can deeply fear it and reject it, just as much as we do with our anxious thoughts and feelings. Somehow we think it is bad to be negative and so we push against it, thereby, ironically, making it stronger. The negative mind is the strongest of the states of mind. It has to be. In conjunction with the amygdala, it is the reason we have survived, as a species, for so long.

We have a curious notion that we should, we ought to, we *must* be positive, and this is exhausting, constantly pushing against how our brains have been wired. In that judgment alone we continually loop back to the negative, never letting go, just in case the worst-case scenario comes to pass.

Once you know the physical signs and the internal thought process, even without an external trigger, you will know you are in the negative mind, because the mind will continue to tunnel, sometimes for days after an event, no matter how small or seemingly pointless it was. Here, again, is the amygdala looking for safety, for resolution.

You have already started an important journey toward conscious awareness. The exercise below is designed to help you go further and build personal awareness of those parts of your day, your life, your story that are likely to take you into the negative mind or activate the sympathetic system. This is helpful because the consciousness that it awakens will then open up the possibility for you to choose to respond differently.

We are going to go to an almost-lost land, the Land of Calm. The internet, phones and the relentless brain hacking and data gathering that you allow to be the norm have robbed you of this place, rendered it invisible.

It is a cruel and hostile landscape that we need to lay bare first. We are going to plot all the trips and traps, the tricks and wiles that are laid for you, and that you, in turn, lay for yourself. We need to know what you are up against!

Think about everything around you that demands attention and where those demands lie. These moments of feeling triggered may take you out of your calm, and sometimes they do need to: the midwife appointment has to happen on time, as do daily tasks like laundry, food shopping, cooking and clearing up. Similarly, there may also be an arc of unnecessary distractions around you that you could learn to notice do not require urgent action and, from there, learn to manage better. Simple things such as making the baby's room perfect all by yourself, a pregnancy group chat that pings messages all the time, your sister constantly getting in touch for updates on your pregnancy, a pregnancy app that buzzes to remind you to check something or a news story about birth or babies.

Take a look through the prompts below, which may help raise your awareness of your triggers:

- **Phone:** Do your eyebrows shoot up or does your throat tighten every time you hear a text notification?
- **Apps:** Does your heart rate increase when you get an alert to tell you that you haven't yet logged your weight?
- **Social media:** Did you linger too long on a sad story about someone else's baby and now all you can see are terrible stories about childbirth that make you feel panicked, frantically clicking through tags, links, profiles, trying to see how someone else's story ends?
- **Messages:** Do you notice that group chat you joined with other pregnant women is constantly making you feel "less than" or worried?

As you raise your awareness, you will begin to pay attention to when you are triggered. Your triggers can lead you to other tricky places—one anxious thought can send you tunneling into others. This is what the brain does, like a line of dominoes falling and the amygdala looking to find safety. All this will have an impact on how your baby responds inside you.

You are going to make a map for yourself of everything that triggers you, everything that takes you out of calm.

Tape two pieces of paper together. Write the words "CALM IN PREGNANCY" in the center and, from there, pick from the possible triggers listed below. It may be that none of my suggestions apply and, if this is the case, you can use the list to kick against and find your own.

Note all the ways in which you are taken out of calm, presence and conscious awareness. You may have answered the three questions on page 64, and in those there is also information to bring in here.

The mind map—for this is what it is, no pun intended—is a tool to raise your own awareness of where you lose agency, drop back into your story, behave unconsciously, get triggered, act reactively and allow external events, and so much more, to disturb your peace of mind.

Possible triggers:

- information overload
- compare and despair
- personal history
- memories
- weight gain
- stretchmarks
- others' opinions
- comments on your body
- people or strangers touching your belly
- clothes
- food
- slowing down
- scans
- medical appointments
- hospital attendance

- labor
- morning sickness
- bone and joint pain
- birth stories
- discomfort in the womb
- endless measuring
- the "shoulds"
- baby weight
- fear of missing out
- crying
- bills
- rent
- lists of all the baby's needs
- anxiety
- loss of sleep
- family
- in-laws
- arguments

When you begin to notice your triggers, you can pull your-self back, use one of the breaths, stretch, sit down and breathe slowly, gently, to reset your system and, smiling as you do, know that this is another conscious choice in the attunement of yourself with your baby.

Remember: sometimes it really is not your circus and they are not your monkeys.

With the tools of stretching and breathwork in Part 2, you will learn to be—to actually *become*—conscious of the shift into the negative mind, and from there choose to manage and change how you feel.

THE POSITIVE MIND

We have a tendency to think the positive mind is the opposite of the negative one, and that it is somehow a much better way to be—always sunny, smiling, seeing the best in everyone. The positive mind wants to dance, charge about being mischievous, laugh with friends.

I am a fan of the positive mind, but it is surprisingly hard to stay there because we will inevitably move over again to the negative: the thrill that comes from inviting everyone you've ever met to a baby shower, but then having to clean up; going on a huge shopping spree after a positive scan and then realizing that nothing you purchased will fit you in a month; deciding you can take on decorating the entire nursery on your own while managing an enormous bump; calling everyone you know to tell them about the birth of your baby and finding yourself on the phone for hours listening to their birth stories instead!

The positive mind is fun, for a while.

Why did I have to add the negative and positive minds to all of the stuff about the stress system? Think of it as shorthand, a shortcut to knowing exactly where you are in thought, feeling and being.

There is another option—the neutral mind. This is where you are when you have agency over your stress system.

THE NEUTRAL MIND

The neutral mind is this hidden space, unknown until we name it. "Neutral" sounds dull, a bit like the color cream in a sad rented apartment, I know. But the neutral mind is far from boring.

This specific mind sits between the negative and positive minds. The neutral mind allows us to ask: *OK, what is this? Am I safe? Can I take time and space to consider my response?* When you come out of the contractions of the negative mind and choose to attune, you can choose to stop for a moment.

The neutral mind is the expansive space you can choose to access through breathwork. It is one of the most exquisite places you can ever get to because it means you have totally and utterly accepted yourself and what is happening. Moving through daily tasks, sitting in the midst of a heated argument or debate, walking in the park, you can be without any judgment or polarity. You will have landed yourself right here, right now: no *pain of the past*, no *fear of the future*, no coloring or trying to control anything. You will reach absolute, complete stillness and, in this, bliss is available to you. In the neutral mind you can stop and smell the roses, watch the ducklings paddle madly to keep up with mommy duck, listen to the rain falling, notice the lovely edge of sunlight catching the sides of the tulips on the windowsill.

The neutral mind is where you are able to sit in this magical space, the eye of the storm, and in that storm create an oasis of calm. You land. You see the madness going on all around you and are able to be still. You know how to attune to how you feel and be neutral; no need to blow up, retort, judge or have a political opinion. It is what it is, now, here.

When you consciously take over the speed, length and timing of your breath, you instantly tell your negative mind that you can manage the situation you are in, that you are the adult and that you are taking over and choosing how you feel.

When we breathe consciously, we slow down our breathing. We choose to do this, to take breaths that are longer, to hold or suspend the breath for a moment. Think back to the breath we did on page 49: five seconds in, hold for a moment, five seconds out. We took your breathing down to five or six times a minute. This is a huge shift from the 15 breaths a minute we can see when the stress system is activated (page 39).

With just this simple change—consciously tuning into the rate of the breath—you told your mind and body that you were safe. Safe enough to slow down your breathing. In turn, this was communicated to the child within, and if another person joined you, this would occur within them, too.

Think of it like this: *You are safe, I am safe, we are safe.*

Interestingly, this slower breathing brings more oxygen into the body and so more is delivered to your placenta. Belly breathing also expands lung capacity, which we'll explore further in Chapter 5.

As you become more used to it, the neutral mind becomes where you want to be. This expansive space is an extraordinary place to be able to take yourself. You can get to a point where everything is peaceful, calm and you really can be still.

If you have any religious or spiritual belief systems, you could consider the neutral mind to be the place where you allow that everything is perfect, that there is a bigger picture. Perhaps it is where you start the journey of learning to trust yourself and discovering that the universe really does have her hand on your back. You could begin to believe that, as you move through this pregnancy and the earliest months after your baby arrives, no matter what happens, everything is exactly as it should be. There is a divine plan. If you can become present in each moment, using the power of your breath, then you will face differently the challenges that may come.

You are sitting after stretching and breathwork. Everything is calm, gentle, expansive. "Ah," you can say, "the neutral mind."

In the next part, we'll explore how you can learn to use breathwork and stretching to release the sympathetic system and move from the negative or positive mind to the neutral. All of these are conscious and aware choices, being able to move from one state to another. This is about attunement, awareness and agency.

PART 2

The Stretches and the Breaths

Chapter 4

The Stretches

Watching you, at 34 weeks pregnant, try to find a way to get up from the low sofa is quite interesting.

"Do you have sciatica?" I ask. You wave a negative with your index finger as you stand upright and do that thing so many do: arching back, one hand splayed out over your sacrum, sighing loudly.

"No," you say. "No sciatica or SPD, thankfully." You walk away to get something you want to show me.

Watching you walk back raises a smile in both of us. "You are almost waddling!" I say, laughing. You laugh self-deprecatingly and tell me, very serious now, how uncomfortable your back is.

"Can I show you something?" I ask. "It is not really part of the book, but I feel it would be mean not to."

"Please! Show me!"

We head to the full-length mirror in the hall, where I ask you to stand in profile, which makes you burst out laughing. "Oh! Look at me! It is so wild what the body can do," you say, running your hands over your bump, entranced by your own largesse.

"Notice how you are standing, how swayed your back is. All the weight of the baby is thrown forward, and your neck too."

Hmmm, yes, you can see.

"Now look at your feet."

This requires you to crane forward to get a glimpse of your toes, way down below. "So? What's important about my feet?"

"When you move around your world in this extended posture, belly forward and feet splayed like this, you are putting all the weight-bearing pressure into the muscles of your lower back. They are tired, overworked and stressed, resulting in backache. This posture also stretches out your stomach muscles, making your back work even harder to hold you."

"OK, tell me more," you say.

"Find your toes again, way down there, and turn the tops of your feet in so the outsides of the feet are parallel to each other."

You laugh. You do your best, and I tell you again, as it is not a familiar way to stand, to really get the outsides of your feet parallel to each other. Eventually, you achieve it and return to your side view in the mirror.

"Oh! What have I done to make my profile look so different? My whole posture is different and there is no pressure on my back. What's changed?"

"By being conscious of walking and standing with your feet turned in like this, you have changed the angle of the pelvic bowl, tilted the pubic bone up, making more space for the baby and putting less stress on the stomach, back and psoas muscles. This, in turn, means that the stomach muscles are now shorter, rather than stretched, and the baby, better held and cushioned, has a good chance of ending up in the right position for labor."

"How did I not know this? Why has no one said?" you ask me, still fascinated by the change, widening your feet and watching your belly distend, turning in the feet and correcting the sway-back or lordosis.

"If you can remember, perhaps leave notes on the bathroom mirror and the fridge to remind yourself. It will become second nature after a few days and will result in a softening of your back discomfort, plus all the other benefits."

"Wow. Thank you. I am going to do this, starting right now!" You turn your face away from the mirror and beam. "You said it would help with the baby's positioning for labor. Is that right?"

"Actually, yes, it can. If you know you want to deliver vaginally, there is another thing worth knowing, and it does make a very real difference."

You turn your whole self to face me, quickly check your toes, adjust and look at me to confirm. I nod, smiling. "Well done."

As you head back toward that lovely, deep, comfortable sofa, I point to the kitchen chairs. "You cannot sit on the sofa now, or lean back in any armchairs."

"Poo!" you say, sweetly. "So what? I have to sit bolt upright all the time? For the next few weeks? I'm not sure I want to know this next bit."

"No, not at all. Turn this chair around and sit on it the wrong way, knees wide, arms resting along the chair back."

You acquiesce and sit perfectly the wrong way in the chair, belly low between your thighs.

"This is interesting," you say, "it does not hurt my back, it releases the tension in my inner thighs and I can see that there is supported space for the baby to move around and get comfortable. Oh! And I can breathe more deeply! So this helps with positioning, too?"

"Yes." I nod. "As does being on all fours, and on your knees, leaning on a large yoga ball if you can get one, for watching TV and reading. Paying attention to how you stand, walk and sit in these last weeks, alongside lying on your left side to sleep, will all optimize fetal positioning for labor."

"Well, who knew?" you say. "Let's play cards …"

To stretch out the body is to release the mind from the bonds of limiting thoughts. By stretching and opening up you make space in the body for the growing baby. And the result of stretching is that your mind becomes still, quiet. From here, breathwork is easier and simpler, because once you sit to breathe, you are already in a neutral place.

As we explored in Chapter 3, to be neutral is to have all bodily functions running as they ought to, at an optimal level for pregnancy. The breath is calm, the heart rate is slow and the hormonal flow is in a state of rest and digest. Your mind and body are no longer running at high speed. As a direct result of stretching, you will feel clearer and able to take on your daily tasks with radiant equanimity. This has an impact on all the pregnancy hormones and thus on the child inside. They feel relaxed, sleepy and peaceful. Until they get hiccups!

Simply put, stretching opens the mind. With regular and repeated soothing of overwhelm, taking time to be peaceful, you will begin to notice that the calm, centered self is a more pleasant and appealing place to be. Studies have shown that, as we learn to recalibrate the mind–body axis, stress states become increasingly unpleasant and noticeable. Please recognize that, with a tall dark history or intense current stress, it will take time and practice to stay in the state of release, or as we have come to know it, the neutral mind (see page 76).

THE BENEFITS OF STRETCHING

Stretching out the four main aspects of the stress system (see page 30) releases you into the parasympathetic system (see page 52). This, over time, facilitates neural plasticity, allows for attunement, helps to create good boundaries, gives you agency and builds resilience. This combination changes your relationship to the *pain of the past and fear of the future.*

One of the benefits of all the stretches I have included is that they will release the vagus nerve through stretching the pelvic floor. The pelvic floor is made up of several crisscrossed muscles in the base of the pelvis. As noted in Chapter 1, you can have a hypertonic (too tight) pelvic floor, which is part of the stress cycle. The movements you will be doing will almost all create a stretching and flexing movement in the base of the pelvis, and the resulting release will also tone this large muscle.

Your midwife may invite you to do Kegel exercises in pregnancy, especially in the build-up to labor. Kegel exercises tone and strengthen the pelvic floor, which will, after a vaginal labor, make it easier to restore good pelvic floor tone because of muscle memory. Remember, your pelvic floor does not hold your baby in your body—it is the cervix that does that.

If you are a medical professional or a yoga teacher, you will be familiar with the word "fascia." This is connective tissue that has only recently been declared the largest organ in the body. There are four main types of fascia: ligaments, cartilage, the covering over the muscles and the fascia that holds the organs in place. It is a hydrated system that plays a role in moving hormones through the body, and it responds to our stress levels by contracting when informed by the sympathetic system or expanding when informed by the parasympathetic side of the system. By stretching, we release, hydrate and invigorate the fascia, creating a softer muscular and organ response.

When flexing back into a slouch or folding forward, lower your chin so that you stretch the spinal column and spinal nerves. When raising up or flexing forward, raise your chin—this stretches and releases the vagus nerve all the way into the pelvis, which, as you now know, releases serotonin. Stretching the front of your body, including the tongue and neck, also releases the escape or mobilization tension in the major muscles (see page 35).

Stretching the back of the body releases the spine, the pelvis, the dorsal muscles and, as above, the mobilized major muscles.

If you are using the arms to stretch tall or wide, include the armpits and pectoral muscles in the movement. Stretching through the armpits helps the lymphatic system to clean itself out. The lymph is responsible, in part, for maintaining a healthy immune system, but the lymph system does not have a "pump"—it moves when we are walking, stretching, doing arm movements, to clear away the stress hormones.

Your breasts lie over the pectoral muscles and stretching into this area also clears the lymph in your chest, is good for the immune system and helps to ease tension across the front of the chest that arises from your growing breasts and from holding the baby to feed.

With twisting stretches, notice that the inner thighs, the adductors and—not so noticeable, but equally important—your psoas are released, too. The intestines are gently massaged, serotonin is released, the diaphragm is stretched and the vagus nerve is reset to a parasympathetic state.

Resetting the entire body through stretching also gives the amygdala a chance to stand down, thus lowering levels of hyper-vigilance and reducing negative thoughts and feelings (see page 37).

All the stretches included in this chapter will work to release these systems.

In the later months of pregnancy, stretching also helps to ease the feelings of compression in the lungs, the digestive system and through the back, as well as easing the muscles underneath your changing breasts.

TOUCH

The sense of touch in pregnancy has not been widely studied beyond the awareness that increased blood flow to the breasts and genitals can make touch welcome or extremely irritating. What has been studied is your baby's sense of touch, which is the first of their senses to develop. There can be an increase in the baby's movements in utero when you touch your abdomen.

Quite often our irritation with touch is linked to our stress system being mobilized. We have other things on our minds than being responsive to touch; our system is ready to take action. Stretching out the four main parts of the sympathetic contraction in the mind and body makes it easier to be available to affection, intimacy and connection in pregnancy.

HOW TO SIT TO STRETCH

When seated cross-legged on the floor, you should try, as much as possible, to have your knees lower than your hip bones. By hip bones I mean the ridges at the top of your pelvis. If you are feeling stiff, or your knees are higher than these bones, you are tensing your adductor muscles. This tension is counterintuitive to the stretching and will lessen the reset you are working toward. Inner thigh tension will tell the stress system that you are uncomfortable, ill at ease, under pressure. When you notice this you can reach for a flat block or a bolster to raise your pelvis (see page 12).

The same concept applies when sitting in a chair. If you are sitting so that you are straining your thighs or psoas (see page 35) to keep the posture (a slight vibration or sense of "holding the legs together" will indicate this), you are triggering the stress system. Unless you are constrained by the discomfort of symphysis pubis dysfunction (see below), sit up straight, knees wide apart, so your belly is forward between the thighs. In sitting with the spine straight the tailbone will be open.

I suggest being barefoot when doing standing stretches as your socks may slip. If you have cold feet, try leg warmers around your ankles.

MUSIC

Whether or not to have music when stretching is a personal choice. Music can be wonderful, relaxing, soothing and compatible with your movements. Or it can be jarring, overwhelming, stressful. Only you will know if it works for you.

I have made suggestions alongside the stretches for pieces of music that can facilitate the speed and rhythm, and enhance the mood. Of course, music is personal and my choices may not be to your taste. If this is the case, have fun discovering what works for you ...

One of my goals for you is that all of the awareness that arises from this reading and physical practice could lead to you taking on a daily routine—one that lands you in presence, and from there impacts how and who you are in your own life. When you learn to attune you will show up kinder, calmer and easier to be with. Music can, for some, be part of this, building the sense of ritual and ceremony that will help to make this time for yourself so special or sacred.

Music from your phone can sound truly awful, so if you can, use headphones or connect to a speaker; it will enhance the experience.

ALBUM SUGGESTIONS

These albums are lovely and can be used to facilitate the time you take for yourself:

- *Passages*, Ravi Shankar and Philip Glass
- *Flood*, Jocelyn Pook
- *Miserere*, Metamorphoses and Vladi Ivanoff
- *Spem in alium*, Thomas Tallis
- *Stabat Mater*, Pergolesi
- *Mind*, M. R. Shajarian and Seventh Soul
- *Shri Durga*, DJ Cheb i Sabbah
- *Lotus Feet*, David Newman
- *Rumi Symphony Project: Untold*, Hafez Nazeri

GETTING STARTED
WITH THE STRETCHES

Your body will constantly change over the 40 weeks of pregnancy, and what is possible at one point may be impossible later.

During pregnancy, levels of the hormone relaxin increase to loosen the ligaments in the pelvis and soften the cervix for labor and delivery. Relaxin also loosens the joints, making them more pliable. Though being flexible is often perceived as a gift in the yoga world, the temptation to push your flexibility now that your joints are looser is not advisable, as you can overstretch and cause injury.

You can also exacerbate back and pelvis issues by pushing yourself too far. In the longer term, post-birth and beyond, pushing too far in pregnancy can cause hypermobility in the joints and ligaments later on, which can lead to chronic issues.

The difficulties that looser joints and ligaments create in pregnancy include the following.

Carpal tunnel and De Quervain's syndrome

Carpal tunnel syndrome is where the median nerve in the hand is compressed in the wrist. There are several symptoms, all uncomfortable, some painful. When stretching with this issue, if you want to put your hands on the floor, use brick-shaped cork blocks (see page 12) and allow your fingers to fold over the edge of the blocks, thus releasing tension in the wrists. This will alleviate a large amount of the discomfort and compression of the wrist ligaments.

De Quervain's syndrome is a similar compression felt in the thumb. If this is an issue for you, the best solution is to reduce mobility by wearing a thumb brace to hold the thumb stationary and limit the pain.

Both of these conditions are normal in pregnancy and will usually resolve postpartum.

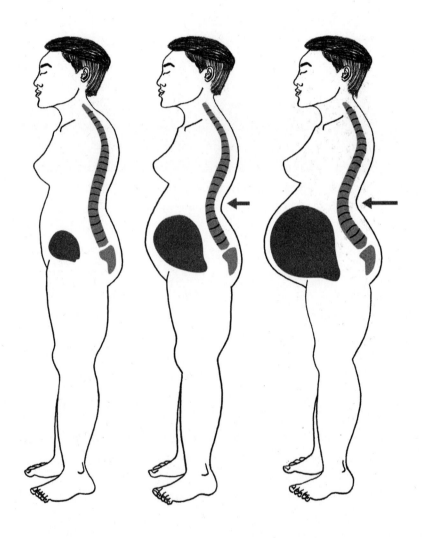

Sciatica

This is where the sciatic nerve is pinched by the sacrum (the bone at the base of your spine, directly above your coccyx, or tailbone), and the pain can be localized to the back or shoot down the leg. It is a common and uncomfortable issue. This can be helped by physiotherapy and by taking care when stretching. It is advisable not to sit on a chair with your legs crossed one over the other at the knee, as this twists and compresses the sacrum further.

Symphysis pubis dysfunction

Symphysis pubis dysfunction (SPD) is often described as a stabbing or wrenching pain in the pubic bone. The pelvis is made up of three bones, with two meeting at a cartilaginous joint in the pubic area. SPD is where this joint moves, and the pain can be disabling when walking, going up and down stairs, standing on one leg, putting on underwear, turning in bed and doing any weight-bearing exercise or movement with the legs apart, such as getting into and out of a car. Doing this may be the first time you notice the discomfort. If severe, you may need crutches to walk.

If you know this is an issue for you, then, when stretching, please do not sit cross-legged and avoid twisting movements. You can still stretch seated on an upright chair. I would suggest that you use a band or scarf to hold your knees together, thus minimizing movement and limiting pain. You need to tell your midwife or health professional about the discomfort so they can give help and advice where needed.

PROPS FOR SPD AND SCIATICA

When stretching or doing breathwork with either SPD or sciatica, you will find it gentler to use an upright chair with good stability. If you have either of these conditions, be kind to your pelvis and do not push yourself by getting up and down from a mat on the floor.

SPD and sciatica are challenging in pregnancy and, when it comes to stretching, there are limitations to the range of movements available. Do not use the floor. On the chair, get your thighs parallel and then restrict their movement by tying a necktie or wide ribbon around them, just above the knees. This does not need to be tight—it is just to remind you to keep your thighs still and parallel, thus reducing the twisting or pivoting in your pelvis.

Backache

Backache is a common symptom of pregnancy and it can be tiring, debilitating and irritating. Only you know how uncomfortable or bad it is, and taking care of your back will come into how you stretch. There are stretches that can relieve this tension, both physically and emotionally, but you need to use your judgment to notice when a stretch is not what you want to do or, in the act of doing it, feels too much.

If your backache is chronic, please do seek professional help.

Swelling

Your hands, feet and ankles will hold fluid in pregnancy. In the normal course of gestation, swelling can feel worse in hot weather and it is relieved by movement such as walking. When sitting, either on a chair or the floor, and not only when using this book, it is helpful to regularly release and stretch out the legs and rotate the feet and wrists. If the swelling is sudden or unbearable in your legs and feet, please do consult your health practitioner.

Limited forward flexing

This describes the effect of the rising uterus on the ability to bend forward. It is often described as feeling like a large stick has been inserted between the base of the sternum (the bone down the center of the ribs) and the pubic bone. Movements that you previously took for granted are now no longer available to you and it is important not to push this limitation. If you are not experiencing sciatic pain or SPD, you can "go round" the baby by stretching your back around and to the side.

By the last few weeks of pregnancy, it can be very funny that you cannot reach your feet while you try to put on your underwear or clip your toenails. Equally, it can be really irritating. How you respond to this experience is a choice!

Center of balance

Pregnancy affects your physical stability. Your sense of your body in space is impacted in various ways as your body changes: you may experience balance issues, risk bumping into things and falling and, in the last trimester, when the growth rate perceptibly increases, misjudging corners and edges. Your mind does not keep up with the swift changes happening to your body and your center of gravity. Taking on embodied practices like stretching can be helpful for encouraging more physical awareness of the pregnant body as it grows.

GETTING UP FROM THE FLOOR

In later pregnancy, the act of getting up from the floor is best achieved by releasing and stretching out the legs, then moving onto one side of the hips and coming up onto all fours. From here, it is easier to rise, and a pole (see page 13) or a nearby sofa will come in very useful.

If you experience any of the issues above, please do read the section on using props (page 10)—they are your friends and will make your life easier.

THE STRETCHES

Prior to breathing, stretching lands you in the here and now, out of the *pain of the past and fear of the future.* A lovely aspect of human nature is that, if you are conscious and rooted in your physical sensations, you cannot think! To stretch is to reset: in the morning, getting yourself mentally prepared for the day; in your new awareness, transforming the awful trigger you have just noticed by choosing to take yourself on; or prior to sleep, allowing the body to release the thinking and emotional load so it is safe enough to go into the night and close the system down into deep and restorative sleep.

When working to calm yourself down, a routine that does all of the above is a valuable tool for transformation and personal growth. As you progress through what is and is not possible in the various options listed below, you may find that you also discover the pleasure in the release.

The selection of stretches is not huge, but they are all individually potent. After each, I have suggested sitting for two minutes in the calm stillness. These two minutes of peace will allow your brain to begin the process of neural plasticity. By taking time in such calm, the brain begins to enjoy this state, to get used to this state, more than the stress states. This is the neural plasticity process (see page 31).

If you wish, you can just stretch and not go on to do the breathwork. But if you can take a few minutes to stretch prior to breathwork, you will already be gentle and present when you sit to breathe. This will amplify the experience of conscious breathing because you will not be using it to come out of the overthinking and stressed mind; you will already have landed in the here and now. My own experience of almost three decades of teaching and personal practice is that I would not choose to do breathwork without the prior reset of stretching.

To help yourself further land into presence and the neutral mind, try to do your stretching routine with your eyes closed, if seated. For some of you, this may be nigh on impossible at first due to hypervigilance in your stress system. The need to constantly check that everything is OK is not something to judge; it is the negative mind in action and it can take many people some time to trust having their eyes closed.

If you tell yourself, out loud, that you are safe enough to close your eyes, it will become second nature over time. Many of the stretches I include here are extremely safe to do with eyes closed as they are seated and require no balance. However, I do advise you keep your eyes open in all standing postures, at least until you are several months post-birth and your center of gravity returns closer to its pre-pregnancy state.

When activating stretches, any of the ones you choose from the list below will give you an opportunity to become more aware of where you are holding tension in your body. From here you will gain maximum stretch and release of the four aspects of the stress system. Everything that you have read and tried out so far will allow you to make the most of stretching to transform your mind, body and baby's state of being.

When you are moving and stretching, try to keep your mental focus on the muscles as you ripple through them.

There are several different ways to stretch described here. Please do take into account backache, sciatica and SPD (see page 91).

THE TRAUMA THERAPIST'S STRETCH

How to sit: *This can be done kneeling, cross-legged or with wide knees on a chair.*

Suitable for weeks: *Suitable at any point on this journey.*

Props: *You may want to sit on a flat block if you are cross-legged.*

Contraindications: *If you have SPD or sciatica, keep your legs parallel with a strap.*

Rhythm/breath: *Twist for 12–15 seconds each side.*

Designed to release all five aspects of the stress system, this is a simple and effective movement to use anywhere, any time you feel the negative mind in play. It also works well if you want to stretch prior to breathwork.

Choose your posture, spine straight.

Interlock your fingers and bring your arms up parallel in front of your chest, palms down.

Create a strong outward tension from the elbows while keeping the fingers clasped, and begin to breathe deeply, slowly raising your chest and hands up in front of you. Raise your chin with your hands still rising, then raise the elbows, stretching up and into the armpits. From there, straighten the arms up, hands still clasped above your head.

Take a deep inhale, stretching up. Twist to one side and slowly, deeply exhale. Keeping arms up high, inhale to the center and exhale while slowly twisting to the other side.

If you can close your eyes, please do. Lower your hands, roll the shoulders and sit gentle and still for a minute or two. You may notice your mind is very quiet and there are curious, releasing sensations in your body.

If you have SPD or sciatica, do not twist: inhale with your arms stretched up, stick your tongue out as far as you can when you get to the top, then lower your hands and be still.

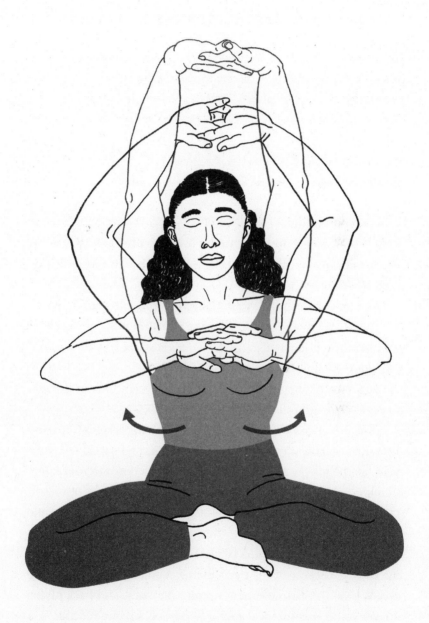

SPINAL FLEXES

How to sit: These can be done kneeling, cross-legged or on a chair.

Suitable for weeks: Suitable at any point on this journey.

Props: You may want to sit on a flat block if cross-legged.

Contraindications: If you have SPD or sciatica, keep your legs parallel using a strap.

Rhythm/breath: Five seconds in, five seconds out.

Suggested music: "Cosmic Raven," Francesca Mountfort.

Choose your posture.

Take a five-second inhale and a five-second exhale. Keep this movement slow and rhythmic. The mind–body axis responds well to this rhythm.

As you inhale, push your belly out and tilt your tailbone forward. Doing so will stretch open the hamstrings and pelvic floor, releasing the tension held there. Lift your chest, raise your chin, and keep your shoulders down and pulled back

As you exhale push back into a deep slouch, tuck in the tail, drop the chin and roll the shoulders forward.

If you feel comfortable enough to take this stretch one step further, raise your arms up and open them, high up above your head, on the inhale, and then bring them back down to your knees on the exhale.

Continue for 3–4 minutes. When you have finished, sit gentle and still for two minutes.

As you progress toward labor this posture will become more challenging because of the rising uterus. At this stage, it is amazing to move the flexing movement up into the chest and back of the shoulders to benefit from the upper-body stretch and release.

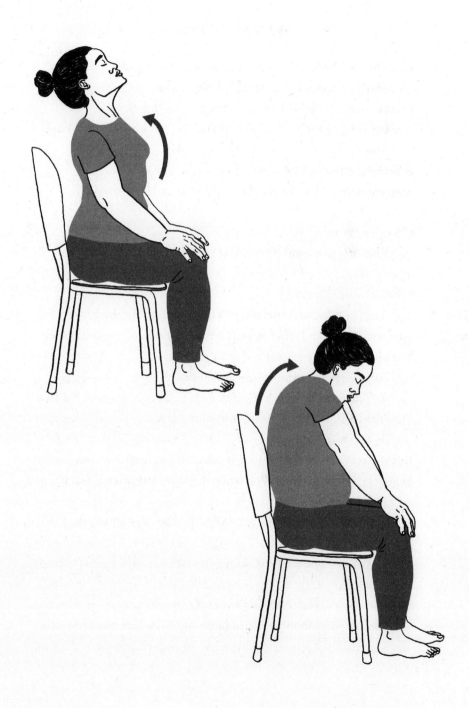

SUFI GRIND

How to sit: This can be done kneeling, cross-legged, with legs straight or with wide knees on a chair. If on a chair, sit toward the forward edge to make sure you have space to flex back.

Suitable for weeks: Suitable at any point on this journey, but as you get closer to labor it can become uncomfortable.

Props: You may want to sit on a flat block if you are cross-legged.

Contraindications: If you have SPD or sciatica, this stretch is not suitable.

Rhythm/breath: Five seconds in, five seconds out.

Suggested music: "Super Chill," Sol Rising.

Choose your posture.

Take a five-second inhale and a five-second exhale. Keep this movement slow and rhythmic. The mind–body axis responds well to this rhythm.

Before you begin, it can be helpful to imagine you are holding a piece of cooked spaghetti vertically in front of you and making it spiral between your fingers. This is what you wish to achieve with your spine, slowly.

To get the movement started, sit with your hands on your knees and push your ribcage across the pelvis to one side. From here, as you inhale, circle your chest, pushing it forward and raising your chin up, pushing the shoulder blades together, around to the front. Then, as you begin to exhale, push around to the back, letting the spine push back into a deep slouch, shoulder blades opening, dropping the chin.

Continue around again as you inhale, pushing the chest forward over your pelvic girdle and around to the other side. You are rotating your ribcage in big circles. Continue going one way for one minute then change the direction for another minute. Change again for 30 seconds and reverse for the last time for another 30 seconds. Spiral up, tall and straight and, as you take the last conscious inhale and exhale, be still, calm and gentle. Allow the breath to regulate itself. Aim to stay this way for two minutes, eyes closed.

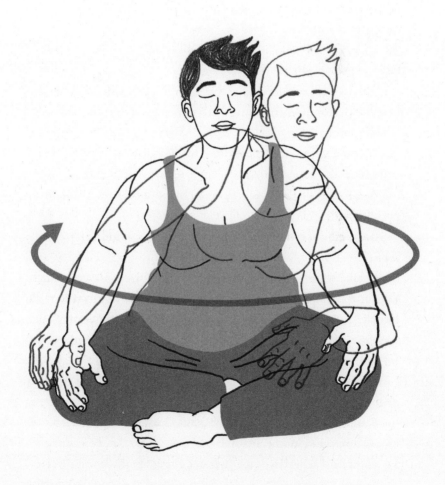

SPINAL TWISTS

How to sit: *This can be done kneeling, cross-legged or with legs parallel on a chair.*

Suitable for weeks: *Suitable at any point on this journey.*

Props: *You may want to sit on a flat block if you are cross-legged.*

Contraindications: *If you have SPD or sciatica, this stretch is not suitable.*

Rhythm/breath: *Five seconds in, five seconds out.*

Suggested music: *"Temptation," Moby.*

Choose your posture.

Take a five-second inhale and a five-second exhale. Keep this movement slow and rhythmic. The mind–body axis responds well to this rhythm.

Sit on a chair or on the floor, ideally with your legs crossed if you are on the floor. Bring your hands up to your shoulders, fingers in front, thumbs behind, elbows wide open. This stretch goes deep into the lungs.

Sit facing forward and take a deep inhale and then exhale. Twist the top of your torso and your head around to the left and, there, take a deep inhale. Carry your full lungs to the right-hand side, turning both the top of your torso and your head to the right. Exhale. Notice as you move across your body with full lungs that you are activating each side of the ribs in a positive, opening way. In essence, you are inhaling left and exhaling right. Take the exhaled torso back across your body to the left side and inhale deeply. Hold the breath as you move to the right again, twisting torso and head to that side, and exhale. Come back to the left with empty lungs and inhale again.

Keep this slow, rhythmic twisting going for three minutes.

Inhale, exhale and be still, calm and gentle. Aim to stay this way for two minutes, eyes closed.

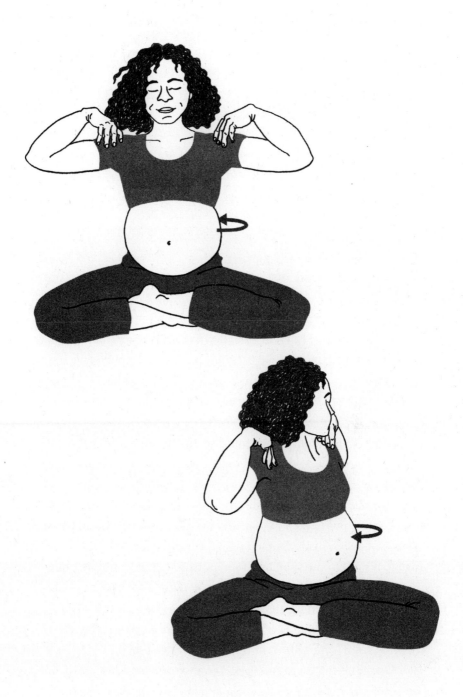

CAT-COW

How to sit: For this you are on all fours.

Suitable for weeks: Suitable at any point on this journey, but as you get closer to labor it can become uncomfortable.

Props: You may want to put blocks under your hands, with fingers folded over the ends of the blocks if you have carpal tunnel syndrome.

Contraindications: If you have SPD or sciatica, this stretch is not suitable. Do not do this once the baby's head has descended.

Rhythm/breath: Five seconds in, five seconds out.

Suggested music: "Global," Bruno Sanfilippo.

This is quite a magical stretch in pregnancy because it allows you to feel the muscles through both the front and the back of your body. It is good for releasing tension in the back and the belly, and in the chest area for releasing tension in the ribs and the shoulders.

Get onto all fours. To take the cow position, deeply inhale into your belly as you imagine lifting up a glorious tail and roll your shoulders back, raising your chin and lowering the center of your back.

As you exhale into the cat position, tuck in the tail, push up the middle of the back, widen the shoulder blades and lower your head, tucking in the chin.

Practice this flexing movement with a five-second inhale through the nose and a five-second exhale out of the nose. Close your eyes once you are familiar with the movement and allow yourself to flow with the spinal movement from tail to head, breathing deeply into the sensation in your body and visualizing the baby being gently rocked up and down in the womb.

Interestingly, this is a good position to work with as labor approaches if your baby is in the posterior position.

Continue for three minutes. When you have finished sit up cross- or straight-legged and stay calm and still for two minutes.

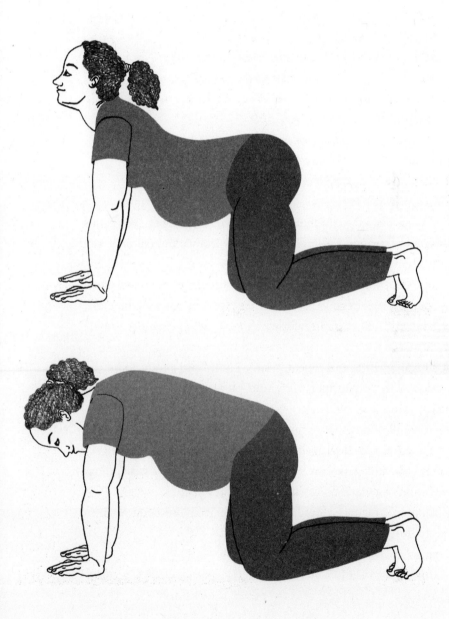

ARM, CHEST AND BACK STRETCHES

How to sit: These can be done kneeling, cross-legged or with wide knees on
   a chair.
Suitable for weeks: Suitable at any point on this journey.
Props: You may want to sit on a flat block if you are cross-legged.
Contraindications: If you have SPD or sciatica, keep your legs parallel
   and be gentle.
Rhythm/breath: Five seconds in, five seconds out.
Suggested music: "Indra's Web," Rena Jones.

Choose your posture.

Take a five-second inhale and a five-second exhale. Keep this movement slow and rhythmic. The mind–body axis responds well to this rhythm.

Sit with your hands on wide knees. Inhale, exhale and when you take the next inhale raise one arm in front of you and then take it up and wide. If you can twist with this stretch, please do. Exhale that arm down.

Change hands and repeat, slowly, kindly and gently, following through with your upper body and pushing the opposite hand against your knee.

You will notice that as you stretch upward the shoulders twist and the hand on the opposite knee will push the inner thigh open. This is good unless you have SPD or sciatica, in which case do not go as wide or as far.

Continue for three minutes. When you have finished stay calm and still for two minutes.

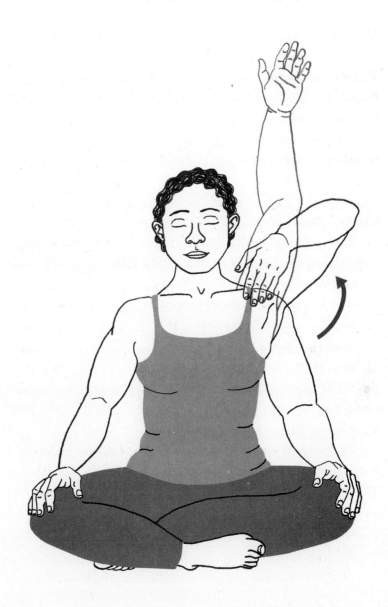

ROLLING THE SHOULDERS

How to sit: This can be done kneeling, cross-legged, with legs straight or with wide knees on a chair.

Suitable for weeks: Suitable at any point on this journey.

Props: You may want to sit on a flat block if you are cross-legged.

Contraindications: None.

Rhythm/breath: Five seconds in, five seconds out.

Suggested music: "Mémoires du futur," René Aubry.

This is a great reset to the stress system at any time.

Choose your posture.

Take a five-second inhale and a five-second exhale. Keep this movement slow and rhythmic. The mind–body axis responds well to this rhythm.

You are going to go deeply into the neck, shoulders, pectoral muscles and upper ribs.

Sitting straight, inhale as you roll your shoulders forward and up. As you exhale, roll the shoulders back and down—big, deep, slow rolls. You might hear curious creaking sounds in your ears; that is OK.

After a minute, alternate the rolling shoulders. First, do a complete roll on one side, then the other, setting up a movement from one side of your upper body to the other.

After a minute or more, inhale both shoulders up high, almost to touch your ears, and on the exhale just let them drop. Inhale up and drop. Continue like this for a further minute.

Then sit and enjoy the stillness for two minutes.

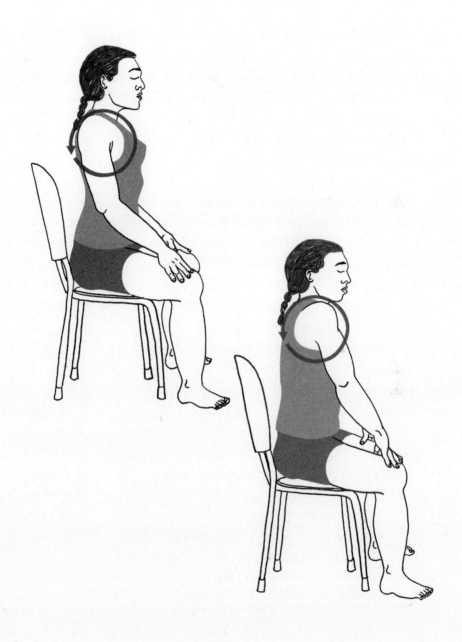

STANDING STRETCHES

How to stand: Stand with your back and pelvis against a wall.
Suitable for weeks: Not suitable after 32 weeks.
Props: Doing this on a yoga mat is best, so your feet do not slip.
Contraindications: This is not suitable if you have SPD or sciatica.
Rhythm/breath: Five seconds in, five seconds out.
Suggested music: "Gajumaru," Yaima.

Stand with your back to the wall, tail tucked in, elbows bent, arms wide, hands up, the wrists and backs of the hands against the wall as if surrendering. Keep your tail in and your arms against the wall and gently, kindly and slowly raise your arms up to vertical. Try to keep your back against the wall all the way up. Only go as high as you can before your belly pushes forward and your back arches out.

Keep this movement slow and rhythmic. Take a five-second inhale and a five-second exhale.

Continue for two minutes.

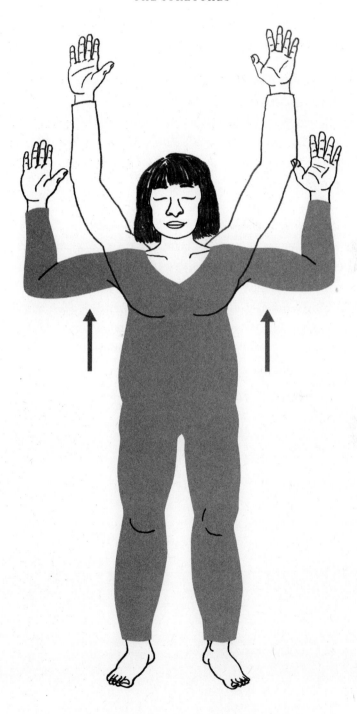

SMALL SIDE-TO-SIDE LUNGES

How to stand: Stand on a yoga mat or barefoot on the floor.
Suitable for weeks: Not suitable after 34 weeks.
Props: Doing this on a yoga mat is best, so your feet do not slip.
Contraindications: This is not suitable if you have SPD or sciatica.
Rhythm/breath: Five seconds in, five seconds out.
Suggested music: "October," Feverkin.

Stand with your legs comfortably wide apart, feet facing forward. Inhale and then, as you exhale, bend one knee. Inhale up and then exhale bending the other knee. Only go as far as you can, and make the movement smaller than you would have pre-pregnancy. This side-to-side lunge is powerful for many reasons, including that it helps to strengthen the major muscles of the lower body that bear most of the extra weight as pregnancy progresses.

Continue for two minutes.

STANDING AND ROTATING THE HIPS

How to stand: Stand on a yoga mat or barefoot on the floor.
Suitable for weeks: Not suitable after 34 weeks.
Props: Doing this on a yoga mat is best, so your feet do not slip.
Contraindications: This is not suitable if you have SPD or sciatica.
Rhythm/breath: Five seconds in, five seconds out.
Suggested music: "Tay Ay," Lamplighter.

Stand with your hands on your hips and begin to slowly and gently circle the hips, leaning slightly forward on the exhale and circling back on the inhale. Continue one way for one minute, then reverse the direction.

This is a little like a standing "Sufi Grind," but the breathing is reversed.

Please be aware that your center of gravity has shifted, so keep your eyes open and be gentle.

Continue for two minutes.

ALTERNATE ARM AND LEG RAISES

How to stand: Stand with your back and pelvis against a wall.
Suitable for weeks: Not suitable after 34 weeks.
Props: Doing this on a yoga mat is best, so your feet do not slip.
Contraindications: This is not suitable if you have SPD or sciatica.
Rhythm/breath: Five seconds in, five seconds out.
Suggested music: "Flip," Beats Antique.

Lean against the wall and alternately raise one arm and the opposite knee high, at the same time. This is a curious stretch, but very lovely in a pregnant body.

Continue alternating for two minutes.

SEQUENCING STRETCHES

Should you wish to create a sequence of stretches by combining several of these stretches together, you can begin to create a personal practice. If this appeals, then shorten the time between each one and stretch out your legs, rotate the ankles and wrists, and then go into the next movement. When you have finished your choice of movements, sit in stillness for at least two minutes.

Chapter 5

The Breaths

The evening sunlight in the room is spectacular, the meal was delicious and we have been playing pick-up sticks.

"Hooray!" you exclaim as your arms fly up in victory. "How did I not know this game?" you ask, tidying up all the pieces. "And how did you win so many times?"

"I loved this game as a child. It seems to have been forgotten now that we have so much else to look at and watch. I love how competitive it is, the focus, the scoring and trying to get the one stick with all those bands on for the high score. I gift this set to you."

"Tell me why you love breathwork so much," you say. It takes a lot of pillows under legs, arms and head for you to get yourself comfortable and I have time to consider my response. You are now lying on your left side like you are posing, looking elegant and very pregnant.

I like the question, which is so rarely asked.

"Breathwork takes me to a place of the deepest calm, to states of being I do not experience in any other way.

"When I sit to breathe I access a profound sense of belonging in this world. I belong in my body, my sense of self expands. I become me, myself, my best self.

"I absolutely know that conscious breathing takes me into the deepest sense of being right here, right now. The world becomes a safe place to be, everything is unfolding around me in perfection and I have nothing to rail against or reject, no thoughts or feelings about anything in my personal life or the outer landscape of the world.

"All my thought processes are still, non-existent, my mind is calm, I am at peace with the world."

I laugh and explain, *"I do not think I am perfect, far from it, but perhaps the breath has allowed me to become perfectly imperfect, and that brings me peace. I do not reject myself or my thoughts because there is only a calm and present unfolding in the moment.*

"Life, being in the world, my relationship with and to the world become softer, easier. Stress and anxiety stand down.

"All is well in my inner and outer world, and when I return from that place to my daily tasks, whatever has to be done or dealt with, I have given my mind and body a gift, a rare gift—time and space."

"Thank you," you say, reaching for a grape.

All breathwork is wonderful. The simplest breath can have such a profound effect in a few sweet minutes.

The practices here are valid and useful, whatever situation, thought, feeling or event has robbed you of a sense of peace. They are also, simply, a pleasure and a positive way to enhance the day. And they are specifically chosen to be useful to a pregnant woman in a stressful time.

In my choice of breaths, I have only chosen those that can be done when pregnant. There are a few breaths where I define the number of weeks at which they are not possible in pregnancy. There is a section on breathwork in the postnatal phase (page 211) that is only to be used once you have given birth, as some of the limitations of pregnancy begin to fall away. I'm sure you'll want to take a peek, but leave these as a treat for later. They are not at all suitable in the pregnancy phase.

Breathwork can also be called pranayama, but that is a specific branch of practice rooted in Hinduism, most of which is not relevant for you, now. We will be using breath in a broader way, and all that is held here is safe for pregnancy, and for your partner and others in your home who may want to join in.

Yoga for pregnancy is an absolutely wonderful way to keep yourself in good physical condition over these months, and if you already have a practice tailored to pregnancy, the breathwork we do here can be considered the icing on the cake!

Your growing uterus causes anatomical changes to the ribcage. As the uterus expands, the diaphragm moves toward the back of the body, up toward the head by as much as an inch and a half. The ribs increase in diameter, making the circumference of your chest wall larger. Despite these changes, the functioning of the diaphragm remains normal—which is lucky for us, with the breath!

BEGINNING WITH THE BREATHS

You may have come to this book early on in your journey or maybe toward the end. You may have started at this point, deciding that the breathing techniques are all you want. If that is the case, I encourage you to dive deeply into the explanation of why we take on endorphin-releasing breaths (page 59)!

Fully respecting that you may have had a breathwork practice prior to becoming pregnant, or have experienced breaths in yoga classes, this chapter provides simple ways to think about how to enhance the breaths.

You may wish to read over, and play with, all the breathwork practices contained within this chapter right away. And why not? It is a playful way to introduce yourself to each one of them. It's likely that, even if you spend only a minute on each, early favorites will emerge.

Once you've sated the need to play, I would advise that you begin with a small commitment. Choose one breath. Commit to practicing it for three minutes once per day. You could make that commitment for a week, a month, a trimester …

My suggestion, once you decide on the breath you want to

explore, is to read through the instructions a few times and practice while reading. When you feel you have understood, put a glass of water by your side, set a timer and close your eyes. Closing your eyes helps with focus; it takes away distractions in your field of vision and, in time, deepens your practice. Pulling the tongue back and pressing it up under the nose, inside the mouth, also helps with focus. This is only possible if your tongue is not involved directly with the chosen breath.

As we discussed in the stretching chapter, it can take time to become comfortable with having closed eyes (see page 95). If this is something you find challenging, do not judge yourself—just smile and notice how strong the urge to open your eyes can be. It can help to tell yourself you are safe enough to close your eyes.

As you sit to breathe, allow yourself to remember that this is considered a sacred practice. You are choosing to give to yourself and your child within, or without (once they are born), a sacred period of time. There are ways to enhance this, and one way is to dim the lights, turn off your phone notifications and sit facing a window. If it is safe enough to do so, if there are no small children or pets around you, light a candle. These are just suggestions, not imperatives.

Early morning is a good time to practice many of these breaths, but we are not all early risers, so find a time that fits in with your average day.

Do note that to take on a three-minute breath practice is not a three-minute commitment. Indeed, I would allow around ten minutes for one breath. This includes time to make a comfortable space, have a stretch, remind yourself of the instructions, do your three minutes and then sit, for just a few minutes afterward, to notice how you feel and to deeply connect with your baby.

If you stick to the commitment, you will be eager to expand on your practice from that point.

The next step may be to add in a few more stretches and an additional three-minute breath. Expand the daily commitment to 20 minutes, perhaps.

During pregnancy, if this is your first child, you may have the time and possibility to sit peacefully to breathe for longer. However, going above 30 minutes per day is unattainable for many of us. No matter how small the commitment, my advice would always be to avoid setting yourself up for failure. Think back to what the positive mind can do!

"I'm going to do six breaths, over an hour, every day" sounds marvelous, and it really would be, but do you genuinely have that much time to spare each and every day? In contrast, a small, manageable commitment will foster confidence, self-esteem and a lovely space in each day for you to bring yourself to a calm space and connect with the baby inside.

During pregnancy, my advice is to become familiar with how breathwork can truly help you; a daily practice is the best way to work.

I will go into more detail on daily practice in the fourth trimester (see page 224), but rest assured that I would never suggest that new mothers task themselves with a burdensome time commitment to breathwork.

With a regular commitment you will memorize some of these practices, perhaps the simpler ones, so that you can choose to turn to them during your day. While you may not want to curl your tongue up into a straw in a meeting at work, practices such as "A Breath to Manage the Mind" (page 134) and "The Resolution Breath" (page 144) can be taken on quite inconspicuously and practiced virtually anywhere.

You can use the breaths in waiting rooms, on public transport, while sitting in meetings … If you feel rising anxiety or tension in a situation, move into a room where you can be alone for a moment and do a minute or two of any of the breaths to reset yourself and tell your baby that you have got them and yourself, and are taking steps, readily and willingly, to soothe you both.

Make a commitment. One breath. Once per day. See where the practice goes from there for you.

Beyond that, befriend the breaths, memorize your favorites and carry them around with you to pull out and use, as tools to soften, at any time over the four trimesters.

Some of the breathing techniques given here will bring you to stillness; others will create a deep sense of peace. Some are so pleasing in their structure that you will be lost in the doing, rather than waiting for the after-effects. Some are energizing and some leave you, *BOOM!*, with such seismic quiet within that there is nothing ... absolutely nothing.

I have given an overview of each breath, as well as the instructions for how to do them, and can only aspire to be a guide rather than give a defining view. Your experience will be subjective and, as I said earlier, will deepen with practice.

EMBRACE THE STILLNESS

There is a word to describe the gift that comes from landing in the now and connecting deep within yourself: *immanence*, a deep and abiding internal relationship to the Divine. By sitting to breathe consciously, and with all the awareness that has come from your earlier reading here, you can begin or deepen your personal journey toward finding immanence.

Sit beautifully. Sit with the intention that you will be present and elegant in that relationship. When the breath is over, stay still. Feel the changes pour through you as the system responds.

After the breath, take two minutes to sit in the afterglow—no phone, just be with yourself and the baby inside. Take time with your mind and body still, with your hormonal flow reset to gentle. It is in this space, after the breathwork, that the magic really does happen. You can go into your womb in your mind's eye and feel deeply connected with the baby inside. Tuning in, post-20 weeks, to the pulse in the artery and to the placenta is also a unique experience of deep connection to your evolving pregnancy (see page 177).

Over three decades of teaching and practicing breathwork, I have come to recognize and know many different states of stillness. In attempting to describe them I not only hit upon the paucity of the English language, but also an awareness that this is subjective. It is what I know for myself.

When I ask clients to describe how they feel at the end of a breath, after two minutes of sitting in the post-breath bliss, I find it delightful that many report similar or exactly the same sensations as I have experienced during the different states of stillness.

I am in love with the breath, with the osmotic relationship between the inhale and the exhale, with the moment when I choose to suspend the breath, with the feeling in my body as my stress system releases and I sit in the afterglow.

Let us start at the very beginning by learning how to breathe.

LONG DEEP BREATHING

Suitable for weeks: *Suitable at any point on this journey.*

You may think that you know how to breathe, but long deep breathing is something that very few of us have been shown how to do. It is a relaxing way to breathe and can be done anywhere.

Long deep breathing is good for aiding restful sleep, raising the oxygen level in the blood, releasing serotonin, resetting the stress system and thus increasing the flow of oxygen and nutrients to your baby inside, as well as for feeding times. It can be done lying on your back on the floor or in bed. However, you should avoid being on your back after 34 weeks unless you are carrying twins, in which case this instruction comes in much earlier.

My suggestion is to aim for 15 deep breaths of 5–10 seconds each way.

Take a deep slow breath and notice:

- Is it all in your chest?
- Has your chest risen?
- Have your ribs widened?
- Is your belly still or did you suck it in?

If the answer is yes to these four questions, then you have just done a "changing room inhale"—this is to say that you have breathed "costally," only into your upper ribcage. We learn to do this to make ourselves look thinner in mirrors or to fit into tight jeans. The diaphragm has automatically tightened and lifted the ribcage. This way of inhaling is counterintuitive to release and renewal. In addition, if you do not allow the belly to expand, you will tend to keep your diaphragm still and tight, limiting lung capacity, which can already feel compromised as you enlarge in gestation.

Long deep breathing asks that you take over the diaphragm and consciously relax it by releasing the belly. When you learn how, the lowering of this huge muscle massages the intestines and releases serotonin. This is called "diaphragmatic breathing." As you inhale, whether through the mouth or the nose, let your belly swell out. The better you sit to breathe, with the spine straight, the easier this is to understand and allow. Releasing the diaphragm is part of releasing the stress system, too. When you inhale into the belly, even at 40+ weeks, the intestines and stomach are massaged, the lung capacity expands and more oxygen is taken into the body.

You may be at a stage in pregnancy where you feel there cannot be space to breathe down there, but give it a try.

Sit beautifully. You can be on the floor or on a chair, hands on your wide knees and elbows locked, back straight. Tilt the chin slightly down. Notice how this posture lifts the thorax and opens the heart center.

You are going to inhale gently and silently through your nose and keep the ribs very still. I know! You can do it—it just takes a moment or two of practice. Try again, deeper this time, really letting the belly expand, keeping the ribs still and pushing the air down lower in the body. Gently tighten the belly again to slowly and silently release the air from the lungs.

The ask here is that the breath is silent. Please do not confuse the "ujjayi" breath with long deep breathing. The ujjayi breath is a specific way to breathe during certain types of dynamic yoga practices, sometimes called "oceanic breath." It is a breath technique that I am not teaching here. Ujjayi asks that you tighten your throat on both the inhale and the exhale. If you can hear your exhale in your throat, like a foggy hissing sound, and you can hear your breath in the back of your nose on an inhale through the nose, it is ujjayi. Instead, try to allow your throat to be relaxed and soft as you breathe.

The exhale reverses this process: the upper chest releases, the ribs slowly compress, then the stomach muscles gently pull in to fully empty the lungs.

Keep repeating this process until the 1-2-3 in and 3-2-1 out feel more natural.

ENHANCING THE BREATH

You can facilitate and enhance diaphragmatic breathing through your posture—by putting your hands on your knees and locking your elbows. You will notice that this raises the ribs and gives more space for your lungs to expand. It may be that your hands and/or arms are involved in the breath you have chosen, in which case you should still be aware of the potency of good posture and its effect on your diaphragm.

Aim to pause for one second at the top and bottom of the breaths to allow the breath to be suspended—no tightening or holding, just an elegant and conscious pause.

You are generally asked to count 5–10 seconds on each of the breaths. Counting helps to focus the mind away from distracting thoughts.

Also notice if you are frowning as you breathe. It can easily happen in the early stages. Frowning is counterintuitive to releasing the stress system. If you are not actively engaged in a tight-lipped breath, try a gentle smile rather than a furrowed brow.

I gave music suggestions in the stretching chapter, but you will notice that there are almost none here in the breathwork section. This is because music can be a distraction from stillness and focus, unless, where indicated by my track suggestions, the music enhances or helps the breath. It is ultimately a personal preference; perhaps try without and from there you can decide what works best for you.

FOR YOU AND THOSE AROUND YOU

Taking on a conscious breathing practice may well lead others in your circle to be curious, to want you to show them; they might wish to take part or, if young, to sit with you and copy what you do. Sharing your breathwork practice is a lovely way to build a different type of intimacy with your partner, family members or friends.

Equally, the non-childbearing partner can feel separate, left out, abandoned in some way. Using breathwork and stretching together can be a connecting experience. Breathing together, sitting in silence, landing in a state of presence can make for a generous relational time.

I fully respect that either or both of you may want to practice alone, and one may have no interest in these practices. It happens and it is not a negative response. But in those moments when there is a divide, be it due to an argument or tension, all the breathwork can be done back to back.

Try sitting spine to spine, adjusting height or posture to accommodate the needs of the one carrying. There is a deep connection to be achieved through the warmth, mutuality and synchronization of breath when experienced sitting back to back.

Choose a breath and agree on the timing. From there, after you have released yourself from the sympathetic system by stretching first, find "comfortable" and gently allow the spinal energy to flow between you both. One of you may be more familiar with or used to the experience of gentle stillness, but it is not a competition. The softer and gentler you can be, the more this will be received by your partner.

Back-to-back breathwork can be a way to make time to be in harmony with your partner during these nine months.

Notice, when practicing with another, if you feel self-conscious at the intrusion, or feel competitive around timings or the length of the breaths you are both managing. It is possible your breathwork partner will fidget and huff, or it might be you doing all the wiggly stuff and, in this, feeling less than.

If competitiveness with another adult comes in, then agree to do the practice separately and to talk about how the chosen breath was for each of you afterward. Consider using boundaries to say: "This time is important to me. I prefer to consciously breathe alone. Can we meet up in 20? After we have both held our own space?" Take the competitive aspect out and make time in the sharing that follows to enjoy the intimacy inherent in talking about how you are feeling, in the calm glow.

All the breaths in this book can be done with kids, friends, partners or lovers.

HOW TO SIT TO BREATHE

You will find that, over the 40 weeks, getting comfortable is not simple, easy or quick, and what you need constantly changes.

At the inception of your journey, the changes are cellular: your breasts are sore, you may feel nauseous, the baby inside is an almost invisible presence and yet so potent a force. Once you feel your baby move, generally at around 20 weeks, you are already halfway through the gestation.

From 20 weeks, the changes are more noticeable: breast tenderness, maybe some pain in the pubic bone, shortness of breath and discomfort in moving; every task can feel herculean.

Your growing child will make demands on your body with their position, kicking, hiccups … I could go on. Maybe you cannot cross your legs. Or perhaps getting down to or up from the floor seems monumental.

If you have dived into the book at this point, there is a section on props and how to use them on page 10. It may help you to read through that and decide how to help yourself be as comfortable sitting upright as you can be.

Then there is the inexorable slope toward labor, whatever that might look like for you. If you know you want a natural or home birth, then how you sit in the last month is also important for the position of the baby.

And so we get to an amazing aspect of the breath: it is sacred, it is wondrous and it can be done anywhere—on the bus, in the car, in bed, on the toilet, in the hospital, while feeding your baby …

Despite this amazing truth, how you sit to breathe, wherever you happen to be, makes a huge difference to the experience.

In showing you how to sit I have no intention of infantilizing you. In fact, my agenda is to be with you in an utterly different way. I hope that together we can create, for you, at every stage of your journey, a deep sense of empowerment.

If you are sitting to breathe, it is important to be aware that, if you are uncomfortable, frowning or sitting in a way that makes your legs shake or puts undue pressure on your thighs, then you are being counterintuitive. As we explored in Chapter 3, your stress system, your negative mind, will be activated by your posture and you will find any breathwork challenging.

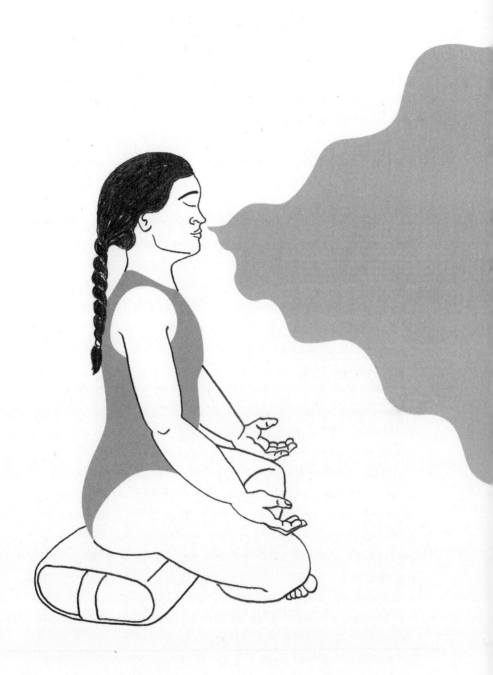

There are several imperatives that will make sitting comfortable so you can gain the most from your choice to breathe consciously.

Put your phone on silent and switch off notifications. You can set a timer to tell you when three, seven or eleven minutes are up. Put the phone aside and face down once you choose to start. Find a peaceful sound, like a cricket chirruping, for an alarm.

Stretch before you breathe (see Chapter 4). This will make such a massive difference to how your mind and body are working and will give you access to the neutral mind and to the spirit aspect of you and your baby.

If you can sit on the floor and choose to do so, I ask that you always make sure your knees are lower than the top ridge of your pelvis. You may need to sit on a large book, a pillow or a bolster to achieve enough lift. Paying attention to this aspect of sitting releases the stress system and facilitates your ability to focus. Sitting this way also releases the diaphragm—this is the large muscle that you use to breathe. You will make more space in the body and allow the lungs a greater depth of air.

If the floor is not for you, choose a dining or desk chair, not a sofa or armchair. Sit up, back straight, knees wide, accommodating your child and your growing belly, and, if comfortable, cross your ankles, with your feet on the floor or a cushion.

Every five minutes or so, especially from 30 weeks onward, please do release your legs and feet to make sure there is movement in your legs and ankles. When you have finished a breath and the relaxation period, stretch them out, rotate your feet and wriggle your toes. You can do the same with your hands and wrists. This releases the fascia and allows the blood and fluid in the extremities to flow more freely.

You may love to sit alone to breathe. You may prefer to be in the middle of the living room, housemates walking past, TV on. I cannot imagine. Please practice the breaths in whatever way you feel is right for you, your body and the baby within you.

THE POUTY BREATH

Suitable for weeks: Suitable at any point on this journey.

This breath is a way of allowing your lips to utterly relax on the exhale through the mouth, with a slight tension in the smile muscles on either side of the lips.

It is a breath that can be done anywhere. Imagine letting go of negative thoughts and feelings as you breathe out.

Sit beautifully. You can be on the floor or a chair, hands on your wide knees and elbows locked, back straight. Tilt the chin slightly down. Notice how this posture lifts the chest and opens the heart center.

The ask is that the breath is silent on the inhale and there is a gentle wind sound on the exhale.

Slowly inhale through the nose and suspend the breath for one second at the top of the inhale, then exhale through pouting lips, slowly and gently.

Aim for 5–10 seconds on both the inhale and the exhale, sitting for 3–5 minutes for the breath and two minutes in the stillness.

SINGLE NOSTRIL BREATHING

Suitable for weeks: Suitable up to 34 weeks pregnant and in the postnatal phase.

This breathing style is ancient, over 5,000 years old and it asks that you breathe through one nostril only.

In this type of breathwork, it is said that breathing through the left nostril only is deeply relaxing. Conversely, right-nostril breathing is energizing.

You can choose to breathe only through the left nostril for your chosen time and then bask in the gentle stillness it evokes, or to

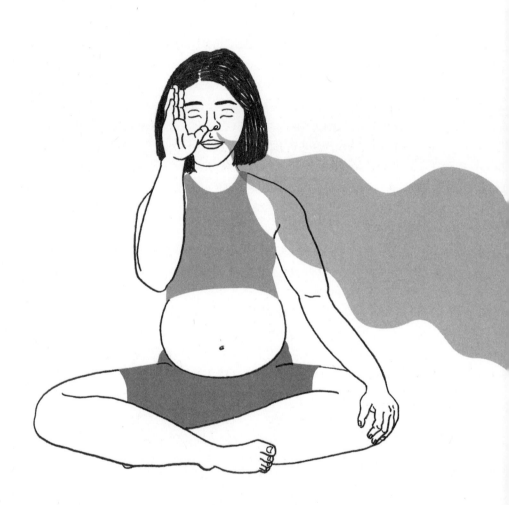

breathe through the right nostril only for the same length of time. Notice the difference between the two sides. It can be quite marked in terms of felt experience. If you need a little boost of energy, breathe on the right side only for a few minutes, be still after and notice that the stillness may be vital, expansive.

Sit beautifully. You can be on the floor or a chair, knees wide, left hand on left knee with the left elbow locked, back straight. Tilt the chin slightly down. Notice how this posture lifts the chest and opens the heart center.

The ask is that the breath is silent. This means you should not tighten your throat on either the inhale or the exhale. The breath wants to be silent unless you have a stuffy nose, in which case you may hear sound in the nasal area but not in the back of the throat.

Close your eyes and bring your tongue back and press it up inside your mouth, under the nose.

Begin on the left side. Your right thumb fits beautifully beneath the right nostril, so gently place it there to close access to the nostril hole, rather than squishing the right side of the nose.

Inhale silently and gently through the left nostril, aiming for a five-second inhale and a five-second exhale.

To breathe through the right side, use your right forefinger to gently block your left nostril and continue to breathe as above, aiming for a five-second inhale and a five-second exhale.

You can do either or both nostrils for at least three minutes each.

When you have finished, sit calm and gentle for at least two minutes.

THE U BREATH

Suitable for weeks: *Suitable up to 34 weeks pregnant and in the postnatal phase.*

This breath technique is a pranayama, so it is an ancient, more than 5,000-year-old practice, rooted in the Hindu art of yoga.

The invitation is that you use this breath to take yourself into a neutral state of being: accepting and allowing, present to what is, centered and gentle. The practice is approached with great respect. It is always done sitting as perfectly as pregnancy allows.

The wisdom states that by alternating from left- to right-nostril breathing you will balance the polarities of the negative and the positive mind, thus taking yourself into the spinal energy of the Internal Divine, the neutral mind (see page 76).

Sit beautifully. You can be on the floor or a chair, knees wide, left hand on left knee with the left elbow locked, back straight. Tilt the chin slightly down. Notice how this posture lifts the chest and opens the heart center.

The ask is that the breath is silent. This means you should not tighten your throat on either the inhale or the exhale. The breath wants to be silent unless you have a stuffy nose, in which case you may hear sound in the nasal area but not in the back of the throat.

Close your eyes and bring your tongue back and press it up inside your mouth, under the nose.

The breath sequence can take a few practices to understand and is shown in the illustration.

You will start by closing the right nostril with your thumb. Inhale slowly and quietly through the left nostril. When you have activated the sequence, always suspend the breath for one second before changing nostril.

Now use your right index finger to close the left nostril and exhale through the right. Then inhale again on the right side. Suspend the

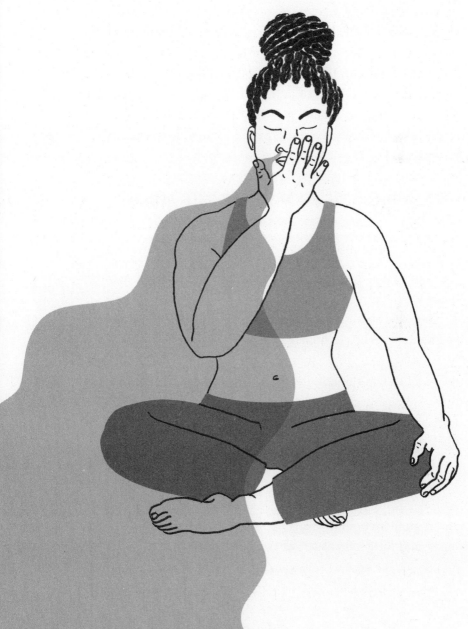

breath for one second and close your right nostril. Exhale slowly on the left, then inhale on the left and hold for one second at the top. Change nostrils. Continue in this way for 5–11 minutes.

To put it very simply, you start the process by inhaling through the left nostril. From there you exhale and inhale on one side, then change nostrils and exhale and inhale on the other, continuing from one side to the other, each a complete breath cycle. Always suspend the breath for one second at the top of the inhale.

My preferred way to sit at the end of this process is with the hands palms up, right hand atop left, gently, in the lap. This is a *mudra*, a hand position, which is said to help keep you in the neutral mind.

A BREATH TO MANAGE THE MIND

Suitable for weeks: Suitable at any point on this journey.

This simple breath releases the mind from the bondage of negative thoughts.

You read about the vagus nerve in Chapter 2 (page 53). When you tighten the lips to inhale, as asked of you here, and slow the breath down to 5–10 seconds each way, you are actively engaging the vagal system through the orbicularis oris muscles that control the signaling aspect of the stress system in the lips. Over repetitions of 3–5 minutes the mind and body move over into the parasympathetic system.

If your mind is being intractable and tricky, ask it to focus on keeping the inhale and the exhale as steady and unwavering as possible. There! You have given your mind a task, which it likes, and from there nothing exists bar the sensation and sound of the inhale and the gentle silence of the exhale.

Notice the cooling sensation of the inhale deep down inside yourself. On the exhale feel the warmth and comfort. Perhaps this feels like a beautiful, soft, gray cashmere blanket that wraps around you each time you release.

Sit comfortably, anywhere that works for you—at your desk, on the bus, on a mat, on a chair—with your eyes closed and your spine straight, chin tipped slightly down.

Begin to inhale through pursed, tight lips—not a whistle but a steady stream of cool air straight down into the belly. Suspend the breath for a moment at the top of the inhale.

Exhale through the nose, and feel the warm, soft blanket of air wrap itself around you. As you settle into the breath, maybe three or four inhales in, begin to make the exhaled breath as silent as possible, and notice that when the breath is silent everything slows down. This is what you want: the slow, gentle, hissing inhale and the warm, silent exhale.

Continue for 3–11 minutes. Then inhale through the nose, exhale and be still, silent and gentle for 2–3 minutes.

A BREATH TO CONQUER SHAMING THE SELF

Suitable for weeks: Suitable at any point on this journey.

Are you becoming more conscious of how mean your mind can be to you?

This breath, combined with a *mudra* (a hand position), invites you to choose to take this self-defeating aspect of your thought processes literally in hand.

In the attributes given through yogic thought, through the energetic specifics of the body, the thumbs represent the ego, the mind of the self. In this breath, the thumbs are both vertical above the folded fingers and it is onto these that you focus your breaths, in and out.

The power of intention is a magical gift, and allowing yourself to blow away negative thoughts on the exhale, and to take in positive thoughts on the inhale, is a conscious choice to change.

Sit beautifully. You can be on the floor or on a chair, with wide knees. Tilt the chin slightly down. Notice how this posture lifts the chest and opens the heart center.

For the *mudra*, bring your hands up as two fists in front of your chest and position them comfortably between your breasts, your forearms at a 45-degree angle to your body. Your hands should be 6–7 inches from your chest. The heels of your hands touch, as do the second and third knuckles. Lift the thumbs to vertical.

When you feel ready and have established the breathing pattern, close your eyes and focus them as though you are looking directly at your thumbs:

- Exhale for five seconds through tight lips.
- Inhale for five seconds through tight lips.
- Exhale for five seconds through the nose.
- Inhale for five seconds through the nose.
- Exhale for five seconds through tight lips.
- Inhale for five seconds through tight lips.
- Exhale for five seconds through the nose.
- Inhale for five seconds through the nose.
- Continue.

You will establish the pattern. I find the easiest way to achieve this is to think, *nose, nose, lips, lips,* swapping the breath each time you get to the inhale.

Aim for 3–5 minutes, and when you have finished, lower the hands and sit gentle and still.

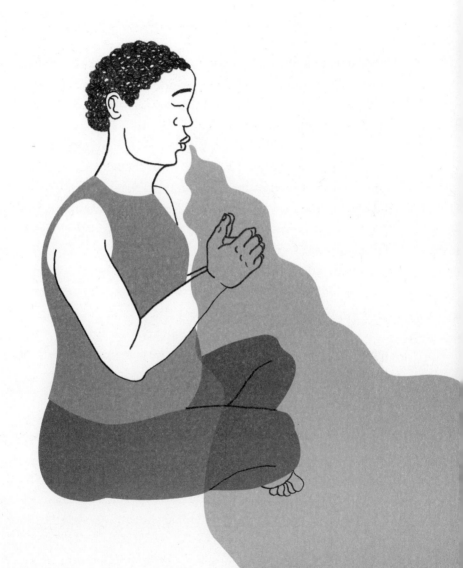

A BREATH TO CLEAR THE NEGATIVE MIND

Suitable for weeks: *Suitable at any point on this journey.*

This breath makes a direct invitation for you to choose to take over the negative mind. This is an act of self-love, to stand down and literally blow away negative thoughts, to clear away the maelstrom of the mind.

You do not need to actively think about your negative thoughts as you breathe—just the decision to change how you feel. Notice the cool breath as you aim it into your open hands. Imagine that this coolness you are holding is a deliberate sensation of relief.

If you are consumed with fears, then yes, take each one and blow it away, knowing that in this choice and at this specified time, sitting, you are letting go, resetting yourself.

Sit comfortably on a mat or a chair, spine straight, chest open, eyes closed.

This breath has a *mudra*: make a cup of your hands with both palms facing up and the outer edge of the hands, along the line of the outside of the little fingers, touching. Almost as though you are holding an open book, your hands are in a position to receive.

Put this open cup at the level of the heart center. Your elbows are relaxed at your sides, forearms at a 45-degree angle and hands about 6–8 inches from the center of your chest.

Close your eyes and visualize looking into the cup of your hands, so that your closed eyes are focused down at a 45-degree angle.

Inhale deeply in 5–10-second steady breaths through the nose and pause for a moment at the top of the inhale.

Exhale through tight lips in a focused stream aimed into your hands.

You will feel the breath go over your hands. Let any negative or persistently distracting thoughts or desires be released out into your hands as you breathe.

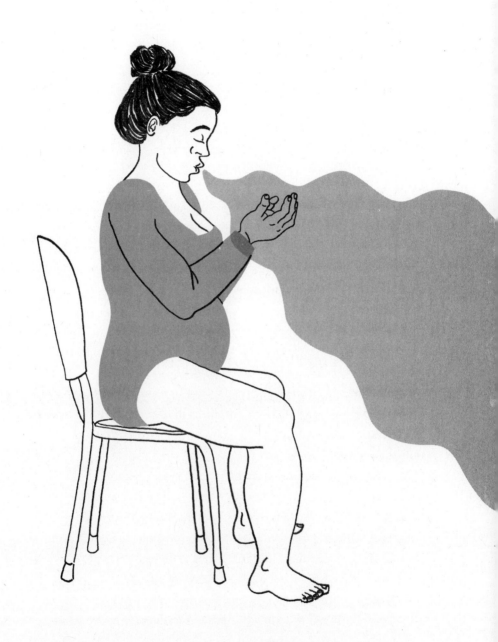

Continue for 3–5 minutes. When finished, you can open your hands out, as if you were pouring all the negativity away, then sit calm and still for two minutes.

When you have finished, roll your shoulders and stretch up and out.

THE WHISTLE INHALE

Suitable for weeks: Suitable at any point on this journey.

This breath is cooling, calming, soothing and softening. And yet it is a breath that you must learn how to do, learn to fall in love with. Not everyone can whistle, and it is unlikely that you have ever been asked to whistle inward. If you cannot whistle, you still want to have your tongue pushed against and behind your lower teeth on the inhale.

Tightening the lips and pushing the tongue forward in this way pulls the vagus nerve and so, at the end of each deep inhale, there is a palpable release into the long and gentle exhale.

Sit beautifully. You can be on the floor or a chair, hands on wide knees and elbows locked, back straight. Tilt the chin slightly down. Notice how this posture lifts the chest and opens the heart center. Close your eyes.

Inhale through pursed lips and make a whistling sound. It is an inhale whistle, a curious sensation when you first learn to do it, but with practice it gets easier. Remember that you can give your mind the task of keeping this sound as steady as possible. You are aiming for a 5–10-second inhale and the same on the exhale.

Hold at the top of the inhale for a moment.

Exhale gently and quietly through the nose.

Continue inhaling with a whistle and exhaling through the nose.

Continue for 3–5 minutes. Sit still in the soft calm for two minutes when finished.

RESETTING THE PINEAL GLAND

Suitable for weeks: *Suitable up to 32 weeks pregnant and in the postnatal phase.*

Perhaps this question will facilitate your awareness, but have you noticed that your intuition is getting stronger as the pregnancy progresses? This is one of the gifts of pregnancy. Intuition is different from anxious and projecting thoughts; it is a sense, deep within the self, that you know whether something is good or not, "right" or "off" for you and your pregnancy. You may feel that you really want to eat steak, even though you have been vegan for ages; this is your body telling you what it needs right now. Or in a yoga posture you may think, *No, this does not feel right to do* and so you do not continue. Again, this is your intuition and you are following its lead.

I love the reality that the pineal gland is in the center of the brain, sitting between the optic nerves; it is said to be the seat of our intuition, our inner teacher. Yet it lies behind the very top of the vagus nerve. This means that our anxiety and projecting fears can feel more real than our internal teacher, our intuition. When we stretch and breathe, releasing the sympathetic system, we can be in concert with this internal guide.

When you are pregnant this gland plays a starring role in your circadian rhythm, raising your melatonin levels during sleep, which has a protective effect on the brain development of your baby, and helping to balance out the oxidative challenges on your own body, too.

Sit beautifully. You can be on the floor or a chair, with wide knees and elbows locked, back straight. Tilt the chin slightly down. Notice how this posture lifts the chest and opens the heart center.

Now lock the tips of the front teeth together. Your eyes are closed and looking down, through closed lids, to the tip of the nose.

The tongue should touch the upper palate, so pull your tongue back and press it up inside the dome of your mouth, underneath your nose.

Project the mantra *I can, I am* out from the third eye (the center of your forehead). Beam it out with focus, slowly repeating *I can, I am* inside, over and over.

The breath will automatically become calm and gentle, soft and slow.

Continue for 3–5 minutes. When you have finished, imagine you can now close your third eye and relax the tongue and jaw.

Sit with your hands open, one atop the other, for 2–3 minutes.

BALANCING THE MIND WITH THE HEART

Suitable for weeks: *Suitable at any point on this journey.*
Contraindications: *If you have carpal tunnel or De Quervain's syndrome (see page 89), this may be painful on the wrists and/or thumbs, so come back to this one in the postnatal period.*

You learned about spinal fluid on page 60. This magical fluid plays many roles in your body, brain and hormonal system. It is said to drain into the lymph nodes in the underarms and into the chest, atop the ribs, where there are also many lymph nodes. This means that part of the potency of this breath lies in clearing and detoxing the body.

When your thumbs are pressed up into the armpits, as is asked here, it is said to balance the negative and positive minds, thus taking you into the neutral mind and a place of accepting and allowing. This is, in many ways, the aim of each and every breath, and having learned about the positive, negative and neutral minds in Chapter 3, this is about holding the intention to soften and soothe yourself and attune with your child. Interestingly, if you

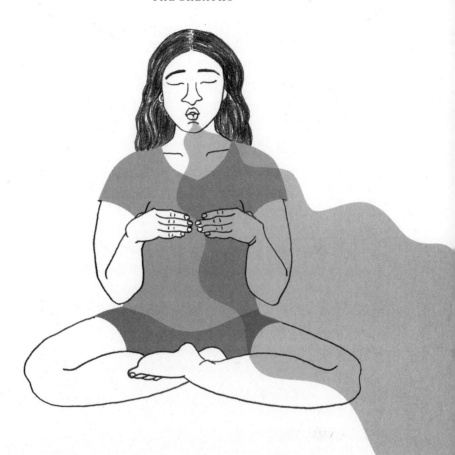

have one blocked or stuffed-up nostril, pressing the thumb up into the armpit in this way will open that nostril.

Balancing the mind with the heart means coming into the neutral mind.

Sit beautifully. You can be on the floor or a chair, with wide knees, back straight. Tilt the chin slightly down. Notice how this posture lifts the chest and opens the heart center.

You are going to place your left thumb under your left armpit, your right thumb under your right armpit. Both hands are open, palms facing your chest, long fingers touching each other. Relax your elbows against your ribs.

Close your eyes and look down your nose, through the eyelids.

This breath asks that you do a slow, tight-lipped whistle inhale, but don't worry if you're not able to do so. A normal inhale through the mouth is fine for this.

Exhale through the nose, gently and slowly.

Aim for a 5–10-second breath with a moment of suspension at the top of the inhale.

Sit breathing in this way, with this *mudra*, for 3–5 minutes. At the end, roll your shoulders and wrists and then sit quiet, neutral and still for 2–3 minutes.

THE RESOLUTION BREATH

Suitable for weeks: *Suitable at any point on this journey.*

"The Resolution Breath" is calming and comforting. It is the hand position, the *mudra*, and the directed breath that allow for the potency of your intention.

Resolve to let this breath make you feel soothed, softened. You are setting an intention and your intention is powerful.

The hands are said to be the external manifestation of the heart energy and they represent how polarized our thinking can be.

You are going to make a small cave with your hands and blow your resolution to be calm into your hands with each exhale.

Sit beautifully. You can be on the floor or a chair, with wide knees and elbows locked, back straight. Tilt the chin slightly down. Notice how this posture lifts the chest and opens the heart center.

With your elbows against your ribcage on each side, bring your hands up, forearms at a 45-degree angle, and curl the fingers of each hand, palms facing each other. Now tuck the non-dominant hand underneath the curl of the dominant hand. You will know which way feels right for you. The cave you are making needs an

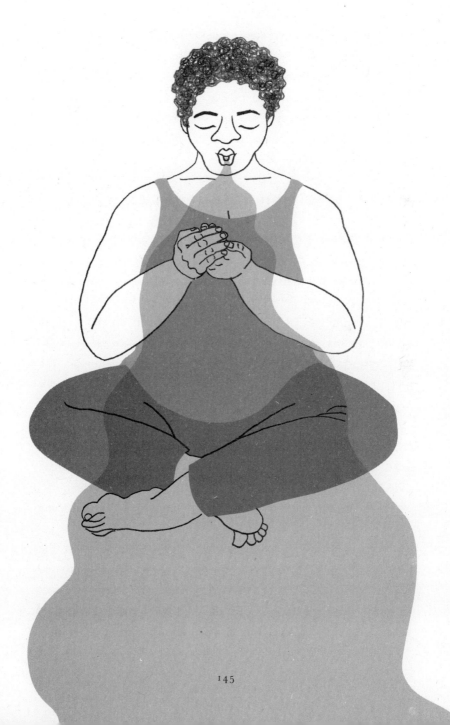

opening, so rest your thumb against your first finger of its own hand, as though they form a portal or doorway on either side of the opening into the cave.

Close your eyes and take a long, deep inhale, 5–10 seconds, in through your nose.

Blow the exhale into the cave within your hands. Feel the cool air swirling around and imagine it is clearing and cleansing.

Continue this way for 3–5 minutes. At the end of the chosen time mentally say *thank you* and relax your hands into your lap, palms up, one atop the other. Sit like this for 2–3 minutes.

THE L BREATH

Suitable for weeks: *Suitable at any point on this journey.*

I learned this technique very early on in my journey to finding stillness. From the first time I did it I was transfixed and stunned by how we really can play with the breath. We have explored all manner of ways in which we are extraordinary, from the ability to be calm and still, to the ways the body changes in pregnancy, to the myriad ways we are more powerful, potent and creative than we believe ourselves to be.

This breath has two specific focus points. One is the crown chakra, which you may have heard of: it is at the very top of the head, at the fontanelle, the part of the skull where four bones meet. The other is the third eye in the center of the forehead.

You can play with your focus and suspend disbelief as you discover this breath.

Sit comfortably, eyes closed. Gently touch the crown chakra at the top of your head. Touch the third eye, then sit with your right hand in your left, hands gently resting in your lap.

With your eyes closed, visualize and tune into the physical sensation of your inhale coming into the brain through the crown chakra. Feel the cool air coming in, feel the slight pulling of the skin of the head. Feel the cool air within the skull. Invite the breath into the pineal gland, in the center of your mind.

Exhale, visualizing and tuning into the physical sensation of the breath leaving through the third eye, between your eyebrows. Feel the warmth against the inner forehead, inside the skull, feel the skin surrounding the third eye pushing slightly.

Practice a few times and you will begin to be aware that this is a powerful breath meditation.

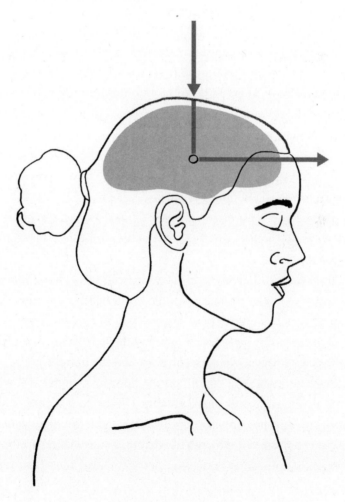

Continue for five minutes, eyes shut. When you have finished, close the crown as you take the last inhale, and as the last exhale leaves, close the third eye. Sit very still for two minutes.

SWAYING WITH THE BREATH

Suitable for weeks: Suitable at any point on this journey.
Contraindications: If you have SPD or sciatica, are pregnant with
    twins, or are more than 30 weeks pregnant, this breath is not for you.
Suggested music: "Memory Gospel," Moby.

This breath creates a mesmerizing, hypnotic experience and ultimately an intimate relationship with the lumbar cerebrospinal fluid pulse (see page 60). This pulse can be felt only when you are in a state of profound stillness and presence. It is one of the first developments in your fetus, too.

I love this breath, as it gently opens up the dorsal muscles, stretches the spinal nervous system and leaves you with a very real sense of presence and magnificence.

To give you an overview of how this works, you are going to stretch out your spine, vertebra by vertebra, from the neck, travelling downward.

Each time you exhale and tilt your head to the side, you will descend one vertebra, inhale up and tilt your head to the other side. Keep your pelvis on the floor and, as you move lower, use your hands or fingertips on the floor to maintain your balance. In pregnancy this is lovely as you are going around the baby.

Sit beautifully. You can be on the floor or a chair, with wide knees and elbows gentle, back straight. Tilt the chin slightly down. Notice how this posture lifts the chest and opens the heart center.

Using a five-second breath in and out, inhale via the nose, and as you exhale through your nose, let your head tilt to one side.

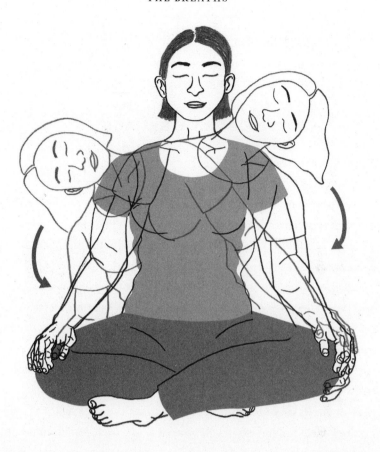

Inhale, bringing your head up to straight again, and on the next exhale tilt your head to the other side. Inhale the head back up to straight. This is the top vertebra stretched.

On the next exhale descend one vertebra lower as you tilt your head, inhale up and do the same on the other side. With each round of the breath, you are descending down the spine, vertebra by vertebra.

Continue inhaling your head up and, with each side-to-side exhale, going another vertebra lower.

Keeping your sit bones firmly on the mat or chair, keep swaying deeper and deeper, either side on the exhale.

After about three minutes begin to come back up again, vertebra by vertebra. Once you arrive at the top, spine straight, inhale and exhale and then sit gentle for 2–3 minutes.

THE STRAW BREATH

Suitable for weeks: *Suitable at any point on this journey.*

To breathe with the tongue extended out from your mouth is an unusual experience, at first. Our tongues are generally quite private or even considered rude—think of sticking your tongue out at someone.

The tongue is a large muscle, and stretching it forward pulls and thus releases and relaxes the vagus nerve. Breaths that focus on releasing tension in the tongue have a deeply relaxing effect on the mind and body.

This breath asks that you roll up the sides of the tongue into a straw protruding between your tight lips. It does not have to be a perfect circle, as your tight lips will contain the roll. Not everyone can roll their tongue, so if you cannot do it, stick your tongue out through tight lips and breathe over it to achieve a similar experience.

This breath is good for nausea, morning sickness, anger and overwhelm, and it does lead to a very lovely sense of having been soothed, in the stillness, once the practice is finished.

Sit beautifully. You can be on the floor or a chair, with wide knees and elbows locked, back straight. Tilt the chin slightly down. Notice how this posture lifts the chest and opens the heart center.

Stick out your tongue in a rolled tube if you can, between highly compressed lips. Inhale through this straw or over the tongue if it is not in a straw. Aim for a 5–10-second inhale. Suspend the breath at the top for a moment, bring in the tongue and exhale for the same length of time, gently and silently through the nose.

Notice how inhaling through the rolled tongue creates a coolness in the internal sense of self and the exhale is warming and kind.

Continue inhaling through the tongue and exhaling through the nose for 3–5 minutes. When you have finished, sit in the cool, still silence for 2–3 minutes.

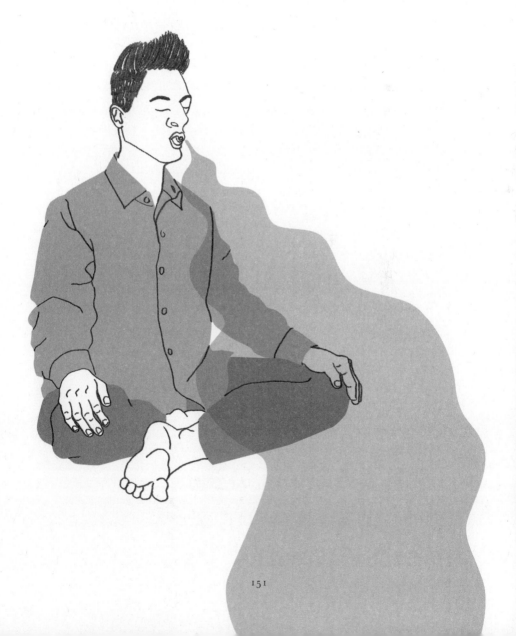

SILENT MEDITATION

Suitable for weeks: *Suitable at any point on this journey.*

This breath reverses "The Straw Breath" as you exhale through a rolled tongue.

The effect of the rolled tongue exhale is warming and calming. The hand posture, with the palms pressed against the center of your chest, is grounding and facilitates a deep sense of being in your body.

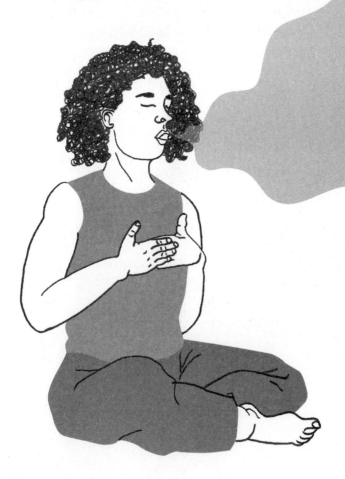

This breath asks that you roll up the sides of the tongue into a straw protruding between your tight lips. It does not have to be a perfect circle, as your tight lips will contain the roll. Not everyone can roll their tongue, so if you cannot do it, stick your tongue out through tight lips and breathe over it to achieve a similar experience.

Sit beautifully. You can be on the floor or on a chair, with wide knees. Tilt the chin slightly down. Notice how this posture lifts the chest and opens the heart center.

Bring your left palm to your chest, horizontal, with the thumb vertical, and place it on your chest with the palm on one side and the fingers over the sternum (the long bone between your ribs). Your right hand goes on top of your left. Your hands are now one atop the other, thumbs up, across the center of your chest. Once in this *mudra*, you may notice it feels curiously perfect.

Close your eyes, lower your chin and inhale for 5–10 seconds through your nose. Suspend the breath at the top for a moment and then exhale for an equal amount of time through the rolled tongue. If you cannot roll your tongue, exhale over your tongue with your lips tight around it.

Continue in this way for 3–5 minutes. Gently, slowly, silently.

When finished, lower your hands into your lap and sit in the silent stillness for 2–3 minutes.

THE LION BREATH

Suitable for weeks: *Suitable at any point on this journey.*

This breath also uses the tongue, which can feel curious at first. "The Lion Breath" is great for anger and for letting go and resetting the mind. Anger is a difficult emotion to hold and an even harder one to release; it can be challenging to find ways to do so that are not upsetting to others. Diving into this breath really does help.

The art is to find the courage to truly use this breath to let go, to move anger. Pushing out a long tongue with the lips pulled back and the teeth bared is the best way. Notice that, at first, you may feel shy or wary of being such a fierce creature. Try a few breaths first and see how it feels to you.

Sit beautifully. You can be on the floor or a chair, with hands on wide knees. Notice how this posture lifts the chest and opens the heart center.

As you inhale, rise up with the breath, raising your chin. Suspend the breath for a moment and then exhale over your tongue, which should be pushed far out, lips wide. There can be a sound like an open-mouthed hissing on this expelling breath. Let that happen, but if it makes you cough, then go more gently. You will find that you naturally lower your head and push forward with this breath.

Continue for 3–5 minutes. When you have finished, inhale, exhale and roll your shoulders. Sometimes emotions may come up; tears can be released. At other times there is a feeling of clear internal space. I do not want to define how you may feel, but always notice what it is like for you.

Sit calm and still for 2–3 minutes.

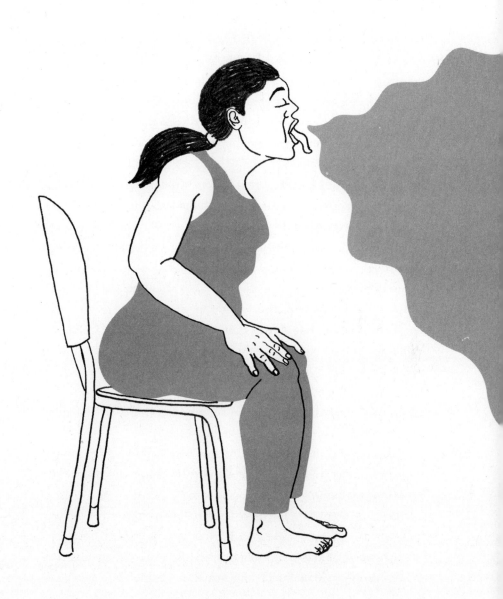

THE CATHEDRAL BREATH

Suitable for weeks: *Suitable at any point on this journey.*
Suggested music: *"De profundis," Arvo Pärt.*

This is a curious name for a breath. When I am teaching this one I also talk it through with a visualization.

Imagine, as you breathe in and out through an open mouth with your arms up, elbows wide in front of your chest (I will explain how later), that you have a huge soaring space inside your chest in place of your lungs and heart.

As you start to breathe, visualize that this space is dark, dimly lit. You can vaguely see yourself in a cathedral, a temple, a synagogue—whatever works for you.

You see yourself sitting on a flagstone or tiled floor and, with each breath, light from a huge stained-glass window high above you begins to illuminate you, one piece of glass at a time. Each breath allows you to see more of this soaring space.

By the end of your chosen time you will see yourself sitting in a glorious pool of light, with the full beauty of this sacred space visible to you.

Sit beautifully. You can be on the floor or a chair, with wide knees, back straight. Tilt the chin slightly down. Notice how this posture lifts the chest and opens the heart center.

Now bring your left forearm, palm down, to be parallel to the floor, in front of your collarbone, about 5–6 inches in front of the base of your throat.

Bring up your right forearm, hand palm down, about 4 inches above the left. So now your hands are one atop the other with space between them, elbows wide. This will not affect your blood pressure as your arms are in line with your heart.

Eyes closed, open your mouth and take a long, slow inhale deep into this cavernous space. Release your belly to allow the diaphragm to drop.

The exhale is the same: slow, through your open mouth. Aim for 5–10 seconds each way.

Continue for 3–6 minutes.

When you have finished, acknowledge the beauty of the space you have seen and been within, and relax your arms.

You will have released endorphins with this breath, so there is a deep and dreamy relaxation to be had for 2–3 minutes after.

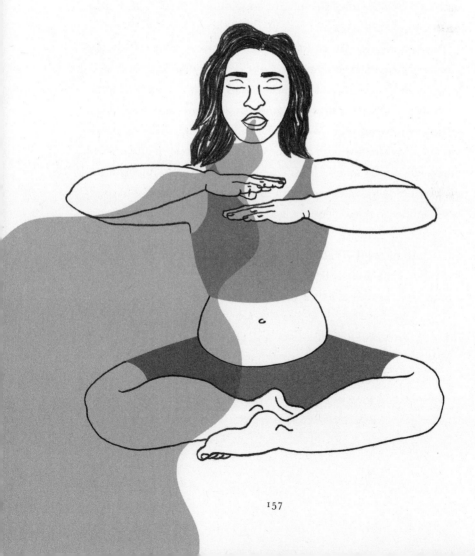

A COOLING BREATH

Suitable for weeks: *Suitable at any point on this journey.*
Contraindications: *If you are experiencing morning sickness, this may trigger the gag reflex, so perhaps wait until the sickness has ended.*

We return to the tongue here for the third or fourth in a series of breaths that engage this aspect of releasing the stress system.

I find this breath deeply satisfying. If you are new to working with your tongue in this way, it can be interesting to focus the mind on the sensations either side of this large muscle and to notice that it never stops moving!

Sit beautifully. You can be on the floor or a chair, with wide knees and elbows locked, back straight. Tilt the chin slightly down. Notice how this posture lifts the chest and opens the heart center.

You are going to stick out your tongue and hold it in place between your teeth, gently. You will close the back of the throat, so you don't breathe through your nose but take the air in and out on either side of your tongue. This is a breath that benefits hugely from a slow pace: 5–10 seconds on both the inhale and the exhale is ideal, so remember to release your belly to facilitate this depth and length of breath.

Continue for 3–5 minutes.

When you have finished, release the tongue back into the cooled mouth and sit in the sense of calm satisfaction for 2–3 minutes.

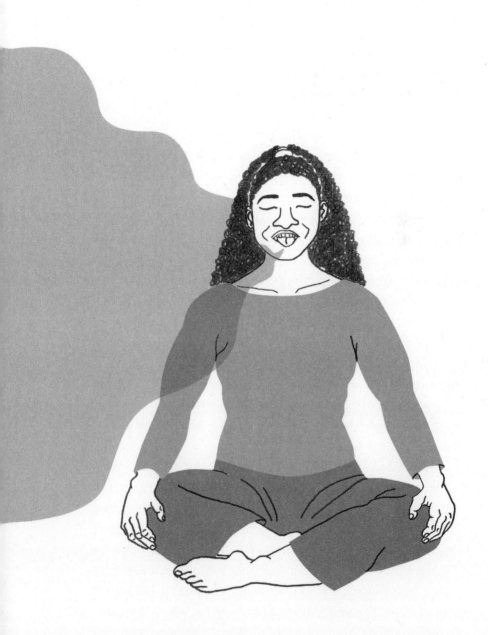

THE WIDE WINGS BREATH

Suitable for weeks: Suitable at any point on this journey.
Suggested music: "Gholame Mosaflenim Delbar," M. R. Shajarian
and Seventh Soul or "Memory Gospel," Moby.

You have discovered so many ways to play with the breath, your intention, the magic of you and the vast realms of possibility that exist in the states of presence. This combination of breathing with movement is a perfect collaboration.

I have written in another breath—"A Breath to Open the Heart" (page 199)—about how the arms are said, in ancient yogic philosophy, to be an extension of the heart energy. An open heart is the opposite to the anxious and constricted sensations we can have when we reject the other to protect ourselves, or when we feel abandoned and childlike.

With this breath meditation your arms will magically become huge wings. Before starting, take a moment to consider what your wings look like, how wide they are and how long the feathers are. Mine are creamy white with gold streaks and dark celestial blue tips. They are 13 feet wide, from tip to tip. When playing with this experience, allow yourself to suspend disbelief and feel the air moving through your wings as you raise and lower your arms with the breath.

As well as taking you into a very particular relationship with yourself, this movement has several physical effects, including releasing tension across the upper chest, which can come from sore breasts or holding the baby to feed. You also open and widen the ribs, thus releasing the intercostal and thoracic muscles and stretching the diaphragm. Lymph is cleared by the up-and-down movement, so it detoxifies stress hormones from your system too.

Sit beautifully. You can be on the floor or a chair, with wide knees. Tilt the chin slightly down. Notice how this posture lifts the chest and opens the heart center.

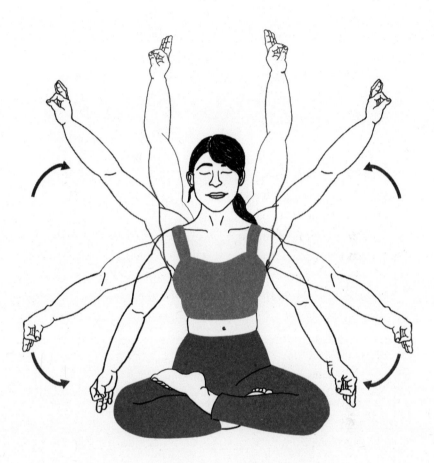

Your hands come into Gyan *mudra*. Your index finger and thumb pads touch on each hand, with the other three fingers straight. Bring your arms down on either side of your body, fingertips touching the mat or either side of the chair. This palm-down hand posture is how you will be at the end of the exhale.

As you take a long, deep, 5–10-second inhale, raise your arms on either side of you. Bring your hands into Gyan *mudra*, back to back, above your head.

Slowly exhaling, again for 5–10 seconds, bring your arms down to either side of you, to the floor or chair.

Continue in this way for as long as you like—I suggest 3–9 minutes—feeling the feathers spread wide open as you breathe in with the arms rising, and focusing on the different sensation as your arms descend.

When you have finished, it is very lovely to relax your hands in your lap and, continuing to suspend disbelief, wrap your wings around yourself to bask in the soft stillness for 2–3 minutes.

My hope is that in the time we spend together, you will find states of being within yourself that are like new landscapes, wondrous times of peace, breaths that make the mind stop and, if needed, help with states of overwhelm.

PART 3

Breathing through the Four Trimesters

Chapter 6

The First Trimester

"Oh my, oh wow, oh my," you say, face in your hands. "My mind is like a washing machine!"

You drop your elbows, forehead leaning on the table.

You say, "I have so many thoughts, things to do, silly stories and random fears all endlessly chasing each other around."

It is hard to hear you talking as you are now, into your sweater, but I think I've got the gist of it.

Raising your head and leaning back, you look at me and say, "It is a spin cycle in my mind!"

We both start laughing. You have crumbs in your hair and jam on your forehead; you do actually look rather silly.

"OK," you say, imperatively. "Come on. Show me something, teach me something. Make this all stop!" And you lie your head back on the table, pretending to sob.

Now it is my turn to be imperative. "Sit up, wipe your face, brush off the crumbs, tie your big fluffy dressing gown around that wondrous belly of yours and let's do two things!

"What is your favorite track at the moment, what music do you like?"

You are now brushed, wrapped up and enthusiastic, looking like a ship in full sail and wearing huge blue sheepskin slippers.

"The speaker is on and this is the track," you say, saluting me. I hadn't mentioned the ship thing but obviously it is in the air.

"Cool, let's go to that wall and take off those slippers or I won't be able to stop laughing. Hold the loud music for now, but that track is perfect."

The energy is funny and silly as I help you get the footwear off. Reaching your feet yourself is no longer an option. I stand beside you and you try to look serious.

"It is great to be laughing," *I say.* "And notice, you are already in a much better place emotionally." *Laughter releases the tension in the body. This book is not actually about laughing, but it is good to know it too is a tool!*

We are going to march on the spot, raising alternate legs and arms. You smile now and tell me that you tried this before and loved it, but when your partner saw you in action it all descended into hilarity.

"Perfect! Music on," *I say.* "Let's go marching." *And we do. Until you are breathless and happy.*

"Great. The spin cycle has stopped. What's next?" *you ask.*

"Turn off the music and the phone and let's breathe. How do you like to sit to breathe? I assume sitting on the floor is an ambition rather than a reality right now?"

"Yup." *You choose a kitchen chair and I join you on another, both of us facing the balcony window.*

"We are going to do the 'Straw Breath.' I think you might enjoy it, given how the stretching went. Can you roll your tongue and stick it out?" *I ask, and you instantly show that you can, very well, actually.*

"Perfect. We are both going to sit here in the kitchen and inhale slowly through our rolled tongues, stuck out like straws, and then exhale through our noses equally slowly. Watch me for two rounds." *You do, smiling at how ridiculous it looks.* "Let's do five minutes." *This raises an eyebrow, but you nod.*

And we do the "Straw Breath." You are slow and gentle. You seem to have your eyes closed when I look your way, and I like that you have not had your phone in your hand since we sat down. I use my watch to time us and we take our last inhale through rolled tongues and then sit, gentle, quiet. The sun comes out from behind a cloud, blessing us on this chilly winter morning. I notice you raise your chin to bask in the warming light. Everything is very lovely.

You take a deep breath after a couple of minutes and open your eyes. "Oh my, oh wow, oh my," *you say.* "That was fun and that was lovely. My mind is still and quiet.

"What shall we do now?" *you ask ...*

There are many different stages of pregnancy. Medically and experientially it is split into three specific stages. I do not cover fertility in this book, so we will begin with the first trimester: the first three months.

Each of us feels our body in our own particular way, and many of us can be well into this trimester before we either find out or truly believe we are carrying a real and established embryo.

In many cultures it is usual to hold back from proclaiming pregnancy to friends and family, other than very close partners and friends, until 12 weeks have passed. It can be in the telling and the ensuing celebration that it becomes more real to you.

Curious sensations in the first few weeks can include a period-like pain as the womb develops. The menstruating womb is the size of a small pear. A fully formed uterus holds over 24 pounds of child, placenta, fluid and newly grown muscle. Yes, muscle—your uterus grows in your body to become an extremely powerful muscle, created over the 40 weeks, to facilitate a natural labor, particularly the phases of opening the cervix and pushing.

Another fact you may not know is that until you actually breast-feed, your breasts are immature. They begin to change and mature almost as soon as pregnancy is established within you, and it is their swelling and soreness that may have been the first sign that you should really believe the pregnancy test.

To be pregnant is a profoundly embodied experience. You have a child, or children, growing inside you. You are taken over, body and mind, senses, sleep and digestion, by this force of nature. A profound sense of nurturing can come in, making you think about what you eat and drink, and of course you wonder, *Who will this child be? How will I parent this new child?*

If you are in a relationship, then it begins to evolve into something else. A third and maybe fourth thus far invisible person makes themselves felt in decisions, sexual intimacy, time and space, and for some there is a deep and abiding fear of loss.

Previous loss (see page 172), the end of the intense process of IVF, sore breasts, morning sickness (see page 170) and exhaustion are all common factors that contribute to making this time feel uncertain and, if this is your first pregnancy, a trifle surreal.

All of these feelings, including cold terror, are normal. It will not feel normal, though. How can so much fear, uncertainty or newness be normal? How can pregnancy be normal? It is in these moments that breathwork can make a huge difference: to learn to calm and soothe the fear, to make it more manageable, to normalize it by accepting that this is how you allow yourself to take a short break from all the turbulent thinking and feeling.

BREATHING THROUGH SCANS

There are lots of reasons why you can be excited by a hospital visit: getting a scan, seeing the baby move on the screen, hearing the heartbeat. Hospitals are, for some, places of safety. You may find it reassuring to know that the experts have their eye on you and how your pregnancy is going. You can talk about any issues you may have and also discuss plans for your labor.

However, for some, hospital visits can be a tense time, and so when attending a routine scan or being invited to participate in a test of some kind, it may be easy for the amygdala (see page 37) to be triggered into visualizing all manner of awfulness.

When hospitals are triggering

As I walk up to the entrance I can see you pacing up and down outside, past the smokers, the wheelchair users and the overflowing trash can.

You catch sight of me and I can see you visibly sighing. You are not thrilled to be here. Walking up, I pull your arm through mine and we head into that curious hinterland of hospital smells, sights and sounds.

The huge, bright blue boards tell us to follow the yellow line on the floor to Maternity. I can feel you pulling closer to me and I gently stop. "Take a moment," I say. You gratefully do. I remind you to stand tall and roll your shoulders back, stretch them wide, take a huge breath wide into your ribcage and raise your chin high.

You do as asked and then smile at me weakly.

"Come on, let's do this. The walk will help ease your stress—let's take it at a decent speed, move some energy." You take my arm again and we head off down endless corridors, passing cleaners, brisk doctors and nurses, empty gurneys waiting in lines and porters pushing those needing to be taken between departments.

There is not a lot to say, and as we see the double doors to Maternity appear at the far end of a long corridor, we slow down automatically.

"Let's stop and catch our breath before going in." Leaning your back against the wall, hands on your knees, head down, you frown and your lips are tight. You are clearly nervous and I understand.

"Let's do it again: take a flexing stretch while supported by the wall, drop your belly and roll your shoulders back as you inhale, raising your chin." You do as invited. I wait until you come back to standing and look at me, trying not to cry. "Stretch up, raise your arms up and then wide, and breathe slowly. We are in the right place, right now. Let's take it all slowly."

We push through the big double doors into a room with yellow walls filled with thank-you pictures and paintings from grateful past attendees.

We have signed in and now we wait. Waiting is not fun, I know, but we are here because you have not felt any movement today and this is the right place to be. You sit in grim silence, hands pressing on your belly, watching the tired magazines flop over the table edge, offering nothing of interest. When your name is called you jump, taken by surprise. "Can you come with me?" you ask me quickly, almost a whisper.

"Of course."

Once we are in the smaller room, you now wearing a blue paper gown, your stress is palpable. I take your hand and suggest a few deep, slow, belly-swelling breaths, which you do and then nod. When the nurse returns you jump again, but this time with a huge smile. "Oh! I felt the baby move! I can feel movement."

It is such a huge relief all round. The scan is done while tears stream down your face and you do not know whether to laugh or cry. The relief of knowing everything is OK has released all the pent-up stress. The nurse finishes, smiles and says everything is good, the baby is a good weight and there is lots of movement now, but please, come back any time you are worried.

Later, sitting in a quiet cafe, you burst into tears and feel embarrassed at being so emotional.

"Oh, having those moments of not knowing is so utterly awful," I say. "I cried too, when the baby moved. I know how tricky it can be, and this release is utterly normal. You will feel shaky and tearful for a while, but just let it be like that. You did really well in slowing down, stretching and breathing."

Tests and scans can lead to more inquiries on the doctor's part. At this point, the mind and body are mobilized, sometimes frozen in terror. (This state of being frozen is part of the stress system, too, containing a sense of panic, pulling in wild terrors and projections.)

You have now begun to understand that you can gain agency over your internal system. Remember the rogue that does all it can to search for danger, for escape solutions and for something or someone to blame for the situation (see page 24)? The breaths help tame that rogue.

There are several other breaths that can be very helpful in these instances, such as "A Breath to Manage the Mind" (page 134).

MORNING SICKNESS

Morning sickness is always awful. It happens as your body's hormones change to accommodate the child within. It can be felt early in the day, but despite its name, you can be taken over by it at any time of the day. Generally, it passes at around 20 weeks, and for some by 16 weeks. Hyperemesis gravidarum—extreme morning sickness—can lead to severe dehydration and will need medical care.

Morning sickness does not happen to everyone, but how much we hate the sensations and rushing to the toilet will intensify those awful feelings. It is clear that no one enjoys nausea, vomiting or morning sickness, but I mentioned earlier that how much we hate how we feel can intensify the negative experience (see page 71). The mind likes to gallop off with the suffering and tunnel madly into negativity.

Recognizing that you will ease the experience if you calm down is an important learning curve. If this is at all helpful, morning sickness is a good marker of an established fetus.

If you are experiencing nausea and an overwhelming desire to vomit, there are some lovely breaths that can really help to make the experience less difficult, mainly by bringing acceptance of what is happening. The breaths won't stop it from happening, but they will mitigate the resistance to what is a natural part of many pregnancies.

Doing a breath like "The Straw Breath" (page 150) may not take away morning sickness, but it will soothe your gloomy response to these unpleasant feelings. And there are other breaths that you may prefer or that will give you relief. "Silent Meditation" (page 152) is deeply soothing and "The Resolution Breath" (page 144) has an intention held within it that will ease the negative mind. Another that could well give you relief is "The Whistle Inhale" (page 140).

In their own way, every one of the breaths can act as a distraction from the displeasure of nausea. The art is to try them out. Even if you do feel absolutely rotten, remember it is the hormones making this sensation and experience within you.

In my last pregnancy, where the morning sickness carried through to full term, the instant my daughter was out of my body the nausea stopped. I did make use of many different breaths and there was relief—certainly I found it.

A HISTORY OF LOSS

If you have experienced previous loss in pregnancy, you may find this has left you with a deep mistrust of your body and the process of pregnancy. Pregnancy loss is one of those experiences that cannot be resolved, in terms of taking away the fear, terror or mistrust, when you get pregnant again.

Let me shed more light on this fear. Previous loss will be a big factor in how you process the entire 40 weeks. If you have been through miscarriage or neonatal loss, then it is undeniable that you will be fearful and mistrusting of the outcome, and that this will persist all the way through. At times this may translate into cold terror, and each time you pee you may well dread seeing blood.

With a history of loss, this pregnancy will be challenging—you may feel doubt, wariness, concern and hypervigilance to fetal movement. Signs of blood, with accompanying memories and projections, will exacerbate the feeling that you are doing it all wrong. All of this is normal, difficult and fraught. The amygdala is on high alert, with good reason (see page 37).

You may be carrying what is termed *a precious* or *rainbow baby*. "Surely all babies are precious?" I hear you assert. These terms refer to babies that arrive after previous losses, such as a miscarriage, ectopic pregnancy or stillbirth. If any of these are part of your history of pregnancy, you may need to undergo extra scans and tests to keep an eye on how you are progressing. Sadly, all of this external concern can add to the anxiety, but for brief moments you may be soothed by expert eyes taking a reassuring look.

If you feel ready to calm down and become gentle, "The Resolution Breath" (page 144) can be practiced with the intention of using the cool air of your exhalation to clear the worries, tension and negative thought patterns your mind wants to tunnel into. If you'd prefer to do something stronger, if you feel a huge amount of physical tension and are getting frustrated with yourself or those around you,

you may wish to turn to "The Lion Breath" (page 154), making a choice to truly move the feelings out of your mind and body and let go with power and with the ferocity of a lioness protecting her cubs.

You may find some of the breath practices that encourage you to be extremely gentle with yourself particularly soothing, and they may help to build trust in yourself and your body. "The U Breath" (page 132) can bring the mind to a place of few thoughts, but also foster an awareness of how incredible your body is—that by breathing in a specific pattern through one nostril and then the other, you can bring such a profound change to how you feel.

Your body, where your baby is growing, is magical, wondrous. "Swaying with the Breath" (page 148) encourages you to use your body to soothe yourself. You sway gently, and you will likely sway your baby to sleep in your body or in the fourth trimester. Indeed, in the swaying motion you soothe yourself. Focus on how gentle you can be with yourself, for yourself.

You may also find solace in "The Wide Wings Breath" (page 160). I would suggest you practice with the intention that you will soar through this pregnancy magnificently. Your body can carry you—you are strong, resilient, capable and choosing to have agency in the process, where previously that agency may have been taken away.

What you can do is gift yourself, and the child within, an agreed length of time each day where you "put it all down" and become still and present with nature, with the gift of now, with what is actually happening in response to the chosen breath and the gentle stillness that you will gradually allow to be there, just for that agreed time each day. Perhaps, after a while, you can have two special moments in the day when you choose to stretch and breathe, to really allow all of you—baby, brain, organs and thoughts—to go into neutral.

Remember that your partner and others around you, friends and family, will be attuned to your fears and previous history. The more care you can take of your emotional health, the more they will feel safe, too.

TO A SINGLE OR LONELY
PREGNANT WOMAN

There can be a multitude of reasons why you are facing pregnancy in this way. It may have been a personal choice, circumstances or something completely unexpected.

In all that you have read thus far, you are learning that, when there is a sense of pressure—internal, external or perceived—the mind can be quite unkind in its thinking. All that you think about in terms of being alone—perhaps not having anyone there at night to talk to in the dark, how you carry yourself, how this will all work out—can lead you into tunnels of thought that are projections linked to the amygdala trying to find safety, and so these thoughts are none too kind. I can imagine that the isolation is felt sharply in moments of exhaustion—when there is no one to bring you a cup of tea, in the daily tasks that relentlessly repeat themselves and are perhaps mainly achieved alone.

Loneliness can arise when there is a sense that no one sees and witnesses, in the quiet moments, how pregnancy is for you. This can be perceived as a lack of empathy or compassion from others and it can then create a feedback loop in your thinking and feeling.

As well as helping to create a special bond between yourself and your baby, the practices contained within this book are all small acts of self-care for you. You consciously choose to reset, recharge and soothe, to take yourself out of any feelings of being isolated and separate. This is important, and the joy of the stretches and breaths contained in these pages is that, for a few delightful minutes, you have actively chosen to look after yourself and your baby. You are taking steps to really enjoy pregnancy and, later, to be with your newborn baby.

To be a single or lonely pregnant woman presents you with the opportunity to dive deeply into all that is offered in this book. Try "The U Breath" (page 132) for its elevating sense of calm centeredness.

There are many delightful and divine conversations to be had with your baby growing inside you. For both my pregnancies I had a small silver ball with chimes in it. As I rolled it over my belly I knew my babies could hear the sweet sound and, once they were born, they recognized the tinkling bell and were soothed by it.

I have worked with single and lonely mothers who made a diary of their pregnancy for the child inside. As the child grew up they loved reading the stories and looking at the pictures.

Chapter 7

The Second Trimester

"That was a good walk. I did not know this park," I reflect, as we sit on a bench in the shade.

"Hmmm," you reply. I glance at you and see that a crossword has absorbed your concentration and you are busily chewing the top of your pen.

"Are you good at those?" I probe and another "Hmmm" comes back. I make one last attempt at conversation with the exact same response, and then I return to my writing, happy to be in companionable silence.

It is a lovely day—kids are charging around, parents with strollers are strolling and talking. I have been absorbed for a while now, forgetting to write, intrigued by a small boy trying to float a boat on the lake with his mother's help. I smile as I watch her hold the back of his dungarees to prevent a disaster. He reaches dangerously far out to push his toy way beyond anyone's reach and she laughs out loud.

This is a perfect way to end a relaxed spring day, sitting in silence, people-watching.

"Oh! Oh! Oh wow!" You make me jump and ask, "Did you solve it? Did you get the last clue?"

"No! Oh, how amazing! I just felt the baby move for the first time. I felt the baby in my womb, like a flutter, a small lurch, like going over a humpbacked hill!"

You are radiant, tears glistening and a huge smile across your face.

"It really is happening. I am pregnant."

"You are."

"Come along," you say, briskly tapping me on my knee. "You are going to get me started on the 'Wide Wings Breath.' I am going to take it on now for 40 days. I feel so happy!"

In the second trimester, there are new changes for you and the growing baby. You will be showing in your physical form—not just the bump, but also for many in weight gain. In this curiously body-conscious world this can be its own strangeness, but many find that it is a relief to be *allowed* to have a belly!

This can be a time of energy, of glowing radiance, and here is another curious fact: you do not lose hair when you are pregnant. Normally we shed around 80 hairs from our head a day. So alongside the glow, you will have shining and abundant locks!

Your breasts are still growing and, with that, becoming quite uncomfortable. From the moment pregnancy is established, your body builds an umbilical artery to the outside of your uterus to feed the placenta. By week 20 and beyond, this can be felt as a pulse, almost like a heartbeat, in your belly. The artery is only there for the duration of the gestation; your body creates it to feed the placenta with oxygen and nutrients for the baby. It is one of the miraculous aspects of pregnancy and little is known about it.

You may also experience what is called Braxton Hicks. These are sensations caused by the uterus building its muscle strength and occasionally testing it by tensing to see how it feels. It is the sensation of the womb tightening for a minute or less. "A Breath to Manage the Mind" (page 134) will help you when you experience this strange and seemingly random tightening of the uterus.

PRACTICING PATIENCE

During the second trimester, it can seem as though not a lot is happening. You may wait impatiently for those first fluttering movements to come into your awareness. They will!

Sleep issues, physical discomfort and the overall mental and physical demands of pregnancy may well contribute to making you impatient and irritable with those around you. Time can feel as though it has slowed down as you count the weeks, and it is easy to wish time away to arrive at the magic moment when you will meet your baby for the first time.

The art of patience is aligned with the neutral mind, accepting and allowing the moment to unfold exactly as it is. Stretches that help with feelings of impatience involve the legs, which can be tense from all they carry, but you may want them to move faster, as if you could pull time toward you. Releasing the pelvis and increasing blood flow to the thighs soothes and softens impatience. "Small Side-to-Side Lunges" (page 112) and "Standing and Rotating the Hips" (page 113) are both good choices here.

If you are aware that your impatience is linked to projecting forward—into what will be, what could be—"Sufi Grind" (page 100) is a good choice that will help you land in the body and connect with the child inside, who is working hard at growing. The rotating motion is soothing for both of you.

WORKING DURING PREGNANCY

Whatever you do as a job—be it highly stressful, standing all day, customer-facing or sitting at a screen crunching data—working while pregnant brings its own challenges.

Nausea can persist into the second trimester. If this comes on while traveling or when you have to be charming, responsive, action-oriented or in charge, your patience can be sorely tested. Try stretching and taking time out of your reactivity to breathe.

The breaths that you choose to help here will likely be informed by the type of work you do. On your journeys to and from work you could take on a practice to land in presence both at the start of your working day and to let go of any negative feelings on your way home. If you are on public transport and are able to sit with your eyes closed, "Resetting the Pineal Gland" (page 141), which employs the mantra *I can, I am,* is an empowering practice to do before facing work.

The news of your pregnancy is likely to have reached colleagues, which may bring shared joy, but your boundaries may also be tested as hands reach for your emerging bump, or as you hear others' pregnancy stories and lots of advice. The "Inner Smile" (page 54) is a useful way to manage this over the weeks.

At the end of your working day, or in moments when you need to reset, use "The Trauma Therapist's Stretch" (page 96), which is inconspicuous enough to be passed off as a big yawning release at your desk. For breathwork, "Balancing the Mind with the Heart" (page 142) is akin to giving yourself a big, kind hug.

HEADACHES

Headaches are common during pregnancy. You have rapidly changing hormone levels and increased blood volume. Stress, fatigue, bad sleep and dehydration can all take their toll.

Headaches can also be brought on by hunger, low blood sugar or dehydration as a result of morning sickness, and a sharp headache may arise in the short term as a result of you putting down a long-term caffeine habit. Headaches may also be linked to excess screen time.

When you notice that time spent on your phone is activating the negative mind and creating stress in your body and mind, step away from the screen and choose a three-minute breath practice to release the stress.

Pregnancy can also create nasal congestion, which may go on to affect the sinuses. If you are experiencing sinus issues, breaths in and out through the nose have the potential for release. "Single Nostril Breathing" (page 129) or "The U Breath" (page 132) will be useful to try. If one or both nostrils are blocked, pressing your flat palm up under the corresponding armpit and closing your arm down over your hand will open one or both nostrils.

Active self-care is key here. Move your body, stretch, hydrate and, of course, breathe consciously. Choose a simple breath practice that is easy to remember, like "A Breath to Manage the Mind" (page 134) or the similarly named but quite different "A Breath to Clear the Negative Mind" (page 139), which offers the opportunity to literally blow stress away.

If you experience bad headaches or a headache that affects your vision in any way, do check in with your midwife or healthcare provider.

BACKACHE

In the introduction to Chapter 4, there is a piece on improving your posture for the relief of the most common forms of pregnancy backache.

As your baby grows—which happens rather rapidly during the second trimester, as they roughly triple in length and become 25–30 times heavier—your center of gravity shifts. Proprioception tells the body that in order to avoid falling forward we should compensate by leaning back, putting excessive pressure on the muscles of the lower back. Paying attention to how you stand can bring relief.

Many of the stretches in this book are wonderful for easing backache. "Cat-Cow" (page 104), "Standing and Rotating the Hips" (page 113) and "Arm, Chest and Back Stretches" (page 106) would be my top three options.

KEEPING ACTIVE

The second trimester is a wonderful time to commit to a daily practice that includes something physical—a proactive choice for optimizing how you will deal with the rigors of childbirth and the fourth trimester.

Create two or three short sequences and then do them on rotation. I encourage you not to make the commitment enormously time-consuming: perhaps choose a seated stretch and a standing stretch, along with a breath, and do each for two to three minutes with a short break between. This will add up to something like a 15-minute daily practice and will serve you well in both body and mind, to meet the demands of, and more fully enjoy, your second trimester and beyond.

At the end of Chapter 4, you will find ways to sequence stretches. The second trimester is a great time to play with this. Your bump is still manageable in terms of movement and flexibility, and for most morning sickness will have subsided and your responsiveness to hormonal changes will have lessened. Energy levels can start to rise and, while the baby is growing rapidly, your center of gravity is still relatively stable, certainly at the start of trimester two.

Staying active has also been shown to help in the prevention of pregnancy-related conditions such as gestational diabetes.

SLEEP

In pregnancy there is a huge amount going on—in your psyche, in your body, deep inside your womb and in the baby—and all this can impact your sleep.

Particularly as you reach the last few weeks, sleep can feel light, tricky and hard to find, and in the second trimester it is not uncommon to have very lucid, lifelike dreams.

Pregnancy changes how you think and feel on multiple levels. This includes projections about the labor: Will you be a "good parent"? Can you breastfeed? Do you want to? With all the stories and others' notions being endlessly rubbed all over you, it is a heady time.

Added to this, as your womb increases in size, so does the pressure on your bladder, so you will have an increased urge to pee and you may get some yeast infections, too.

As we touched on on page 89, relaxin causes all your joints to soften and this hormonal effect is most commonly felt in the pelvic girdle. It is when you lie down to sleep that you can notice aches in the hip joints and the legs.

Your baby may not want to go to sleep when you do and may be awake while you are asleep. Waking up to being kicked inside is a novel experience and does make sleep more challenging.

However, you can gain agency over your sleep. Below are known tips to create good sleep patterns in pregnancy.

If you are still having the occasional cup of tea or coffee, it's best to limit caffeine to the morning and ensure you are having no more than 200 milligrams per day. (A typical latte contains 128 milligrams of caffeine.) This ubiquitous substance takes 12 hours to leave the body and is present in black tea, green tea, coffee and many fizzy drinks. Taking down caffeine levels can trigger a nasty headache for a day, yet once that hurdle is crossed the positive effect on sleep is very noticeable and you will no longer be sharing caffeine with your baby.

The color of your screen, computer, tablet and phone also affects sleep—they all give out blue light, which is in the daylight spectrum and so at night will sustain wakefulness. But all of these machines now have the ability, in the display and brightness function, to move to warmer light once the sun goes down. You can set this to happen automatically. If you are looking at any of these screens in the three hours before bed, and you have not set this function, you are communicating to your circadian rhythm that it is not time to sleep—it is still daylight! Thus, the hormones that want to slow you down physically and mentally, to go to sleep, particularly in gestation, are reset to wakefulness.

What you watch at night can also trigger stress functions, mobilization, projection and memories, all of which are counterintuitive to sleep, and when you are pregnant, violence is the last thing you want to have your amygdala contemplating. If it is in your nature to like horror films, murder mysteries or violent action movies, try saving up a watch list for after the fourth trimester! A good book, preferably not a stressful one, will relax the body into sleep, and sleep is where wondrous growth can take place in your womb.

Inevitably, you are going to want to pee in the night. When roused by this need, don't put on the bright bathroom light, as this will wake you up. Instead use a dim nightlight in the hall to guide your way. Once back in bed, throw off the covers, have a stretch and, when you've cooled down—which will reset the sleep hormones—cover back up. If you are noticing pelvic or hip pain, putting pillows under your knees is a good way to balance out any discomfort.

As you try to get to sleep, for every thought that comes, good or mean, mentally say *yes, yes, yes* … and sleep will roll back over you.

Sleeping deeply is the opposite to being mobilized. To take this one step further—because now you understand what the vagus nerve does in mobilization—to sleep deeply is to relax the vagus nerve.

Stretching now becomes a very effective pre-sleep tool to release the sympathetic system. Stretching releases the vagus nerve and tells your system it is safe enough to sleep. If you can sit cross-legged or with your knees wide apart on the edge of the bed, try "The Trauma Therapist's Stretch" (page 96) three times, slowly, and then bask in the gentle, mind-softening stillness that the serotonin release brings. This stretch will also soothe a wide-awake and kicking baby in your belly.

If you find yourself, in the second trimester and beyond, in warmer than average temperatures, feeling hot and stifled will be a hindrance to sleep. If you find yourself feeling restless and over-heated in the night, "The Straw Breath" (page 150) could be a welcome companion to your late-night discomfort.

A breath that cools and soothes in equal measure is "Resetting the Pineal Gland" (page 141). Given the pineal gland's role in regulating your circadian rhythm, holding the intention that this practice really will soften you to sleep is potent. With the release of tension created through your teeth coming together, and the affirmative mantra *I can, I am*, this is a breath practice that can truly help to change how you think, feel and, from there, sleep.

A final option, well known in yogic circles as a go-to breath for sleep, is "Single Nostril Breathing" (page 129). Please note that, for relaxing into sleep, you want to breathe through the left nostril only. The left nostril is said to take you into parasympathetic response, signaling to the mind that you're safe enough to rest. By contrast, it is said that activating the right nostril will help take you into the positive mind, excited and ready to go—not what you want before bed, perhaps!

With all that said, sometimes, when pregnant, a bad night of sleep is unavoidable. If you're awake extremely early or cannot get back to sleep in the night, using the breaths as a comfort (rather than, for example, your phone) will make you feel more positive about things, about yourself and about how excellent you are at active self-care.

Chapter 8

The Third Trimester

You throw open the door to me with a huge smile on your face.

"How delightful!" I say as I watch you do a little dance, belly swaying, arms up. You laugh and with a sweeping gesture invite me to sit at the table, which is laden with a lovely summer breakfast.

You are eager to talk and you finally sit down with a flourish, lifting your phone and pointedly inviting me to watch you put it on silent and place it face down at the far end of the table. I nod, smiling. I am impressed.

"I did the 'Pouty Breath' last night and this morning!"

This makes me laugh out loud. "Is that what we call it?" I ask, and yes, you affirm, it is.

"And," you continue with great pride, "I stretched last night and this morning and it makes me feel so good." You lean forward, almost in confidence, to explain how much more space it gives you to breathe and how it does, actually, change how you think. And the final offer: you did not get angry last night at all. Oh, and you did not look at your phone until 9 a.m. And ... you have made an agreement with yourself only to look at social media once a day.

"Well, hooray!" I am deeply impressed and you beam anew and pop a plump raspberry into your mouth.

As you progress toward the third trimester, and certainly by the end of pregnancy, you will have up to 45 percent more blood in your body. This contributes to the sense of breathlessness and, as the top of the uterus—the fundus—pushes up toward your diaphragm, your intestines will be squished and compressed.

Your lung capacity is reduced by between 10 and 20 percent at full term. The increase in size of the ribcage is thought to allow the vital capacity (the total amount of air exhaled after maximal inhalation) to remain unchanged, and the lung capacity only decreases a small amount by the end of the third trimester, despite how it can feel.

Your uterus may lower as your baby's head moves into the pelvis before delivery, and this can alleviate any sense of breathlessness, but it will also increase your desire to pee.

Also, magically, your heart turns on its side and moves into the center of your chest to allow your left lung, which is always smaller, to have more breathing space. Our bodies really are amazing!

However, they can also become rather unwieldy at this stage of pregnancy. Your bump gets in the way and your joints become looser due to the hormone relaxin preparing you for labor; all of this can cause backache, sciatica, SPD, carpal tunnel and other bone and joint symptoms (see pages 89–92) that may mean movements including sitting, standing, traveling in cars, buses, trains and subways become an ordeal in themselves.

All of the above—and so much more in terms of cellular changes, surges of hormones leading to intense emotions, memories and your longer-term thoughts and goals for the child—make this a heady time.

There are ways to create more of a sense of space in your internal systems. You will achieve this through specific stretches and through breaths that open up the ribs and their muscles. Long deep breathing (as described on page 121) can be a good way to stretch and release the diaphragm and open up the ribs. Try doing some standing stretches before you breathe and you will notice your body has more space and the mind is still.

In the last weeks of gestation you can also experience restless legs syndrome, where the legs seem to take on a life of their own.

Reducing caffeine intake and doing good stretches will help this, alongside cooling you down when you are too warm in bed.

If you know you want to go into labor—a curious statement, I know, but you may be planning to have a caesarean, elective or medically assigned—then in the last six weeks it is important to lie on your left side at night. For a labor to proceed with the least intervention, the baby should ideally be head down with their spine to your left side. This specific positioning allows the bones of the baby's skull to positively affect the opening of the cervix once pre-labor starts.

Hypoxemia (low levels of oxygen in the blood) can happen when you are lying on your back. This is generally experienced in the later stages of pregnancy unless you are carrying twins, in which case it can occur earlier. This is another reason why pregnant women are given the recommendation to sleep on their left side.

You may never have lain on your left; you may be an on-your-back or on-your-stomach sleeper, but neither of these are options in the later stages. On your back, the uterine pressure on the vena cava (a vein that carries blood back to the heart from the organs) suppresses blood flow to the placenta. There is an automatic mechanism within all pregnancies to make this an unwanted position. You will notice a need to move away from lying on the back in later pregnancy to protect the baby.

Using long pillows specially crafted for pregnancy and breastfeeding under your elbow and knee will help you to adjust to this new sleep posture and will ease the discomfort of breast changes.

BED REST IN PREGNANCY

If you have been prescribed partial or complete bed rest in pregnancy by your health professional, this can take various forms. You will know why this has come about and, if complete bed rest is required, then you will be restricted to walking only to use the bathroom.

Partial bed rest will limit you leaving the house. Your exercise will be restricted and ideally, you will spend less time vertical. However, you can sit up in bed.

This period may be weeks or months and it is trying, to say the least. You will be given instructions as you get closer to the birth, including not lying on your back and making sure you move your legs and stretch your feet to reduce the likelihood of deep vein thrombosis.

I have included a section on stretching in bed rest below, and I hope this will give you a welcome break from feeling bored, irritated and resentful.

Some of the breaths in Chapter 5 can be done lying down and, if you are confined to sitting in bed, the props section (page 10) will be useful to help you get the most from your practice. Try "A Breath to Manage the Mind" (page 134); this soothes a restless sense of self surprisingly quickly. "Silent Meditation" (page 152) is also deeply relaxing and soothing.

BED REST STRETCHES

How to lie: Lying flat is good, with no bedding over you.

How to sit: If you can sit, aim to be as upright as possible; consider pillows behind your back or sit on the edge of the bed.

Suitable for weeks: Up to week 40.

Props: Pillows behind the lower back if sitting up in bed or on the edge of the bed is an issue.

Contraindications: Pay attention to the twists if you have SPD or sciatica. Use a belt or tie around the legs to limit movement but not circulation.

Rhythm/breath: Aim for five seconds in, five seconds out.

Suggested music: "Caro Nome," Maria Callas.

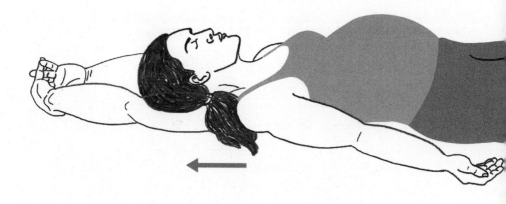

Lying on your back—provided you are not over 34 weeks, as this will press on the vena cava—push yourself low down on the bed so you can raise your arms above your head without hitting the headboard or the wall. Remove the bedcovers.

Raise your arms above your head so they are lying on the bed. Bring your elbows wide apart, with your hands clasped not behind your head, but above it on the bed. Push the elbows back and wide and move your chest and ribcage, aiming to feel the armpits stretch and the ribs move. This will release the intercostal muscles.

Continue for one minute.

From there, put both arms alongside your body, take one arm diagonally across your torso and then raise it up across your head and widen it out to the opposite side. Take gentle, five-second breaths as you inhale across and wide. Exhale as your arm comes back down to your side. Remember to keep your eyes closed if you can.

You can do alternate arms or several stretches on one side and then repeat on the other side.

Continue for one minute each side or two minutes alternating from side to side.

Lie on your left side after the stretches, or on your back with pillows under your knees, for two minutes.

EXPECTATIONS OF LABOR

You may have decided that you want a natural labor, or this may not be a possibility for you, or you may have decided you do not want this for many reasons—some medical, others personal. Perhaps you want a midwife-led hospital labor, and it is possible that you may need to be induced.

In any case—natural, medically assisted or caesarean birth—events do not always unfurl according to your best-laid plans. It helps to recognize that this is not your labor; you had yours when you were born. This labor belongs to your child, even though you are the one who will bear and channel them.

While aiming for a natural labor can be a wonderful thing, I would encourage you not to let that quest define your entire experience of pregnancy, birth and your feelings about birth in the postnatal phase. In a way, letting go of the need for the event to be perfect, to go exactly as planned, can help you to accept medical expertise, whether at home or in hospital. If you give birth to a healthy baby, safely, you will have won the lottery of life.

One specific form of training that you can do in the last three months of your pregnancy is hypnobirthing. In this you will learn how to breathe in labor and the pushing phase. I want to be clear that, in sharing breath techniques for pregnancy and the postnatal period, I do not teach hypnobirthing.

BREATHS TO PREPARE FOR LABOR

In the build-up to labor, the third trimester, there is much we can do together, with breath and arm work combined, to facilitate your ability to work with your hormonal flow. The breaths below are specifically for the last trimester. These breaths are not to be used in actual labor—you will not need them. Your contractions will naturally release endorphins and you will learn, in practicing the breaths given below, how to make the most of this wonderful hormone.

The breaths below could be described as meditations on bearing discomfort. Sometimes you could say they are painful—I know! But these breaths have been chosen because they will encourage you to discover quite how strong you really are. We—those of us who can carry children—are much stronger in our ability to hold and bear physical discomfort in our nervous system than men, and it is a gift that we do not really get to activate until we are pregnant and want a natural labor.

The purpose of these breaths is to trigger the release of endorphins (see page 42). As a reminder, this hormone is a natural painkiller produced by your body as a thank-you for your effort and exertion. This specific area of breathwork helps you to learn to trust that your body can and will produce endorphins. We will be using this release to facilitate your progress through the contractions of natural labor.

Having a regular practice of releasing endorphins will teach you that you can bear much, much more than you previously thought you could. You will learn to trust yourself and your body to support you. You will discover that these hormones create an altered state within you, a dreamy state of being. You can then easily recognize this state in natural labor because you will have become familiar with it in your practice.

When you are in the second stage of labor, the art will be to keep the lights as low as possible and to minimize the number of questions put to you about sugar in your tea or where the towels are kept. If you like music, choose soft and dreamy tracks. Making a labor playlist can create a lovely memory for later. Both my children were born to the same track by Brahms. If your labor is at home, your midwives will be familiar with these asks and they will know how potent endorphins are in facilitating your labor progression.

You can do these breaths for up to 11 minutes. At first this will seem impossible, but it is not. You are so much more powerful than you imagine.

Try to practice with your eyes closed as this will increase your focus.

In the relaxation phase, after your practice, you will always be invited to be still and gentle, to allow you to gain an awareness of how that feeling is calming, almost overtaking. Make sure you are warm and comfortable. Consciously allow yourself to flow with the relaxation after each session. Notice how your body meets your effort and gifts you this wonderful treat, this naturally released and internally produced form of morphine.

I have added music choices where appropriate.

Once your contractions are established in a natural labor, there will be a moment between each one where you can take a long deep breath for the baby. To consciously breathe deeply through the nose, deep into the belly, sends a loving wave of oxygen to both you and your baby. It is a profound way to stay connected with them throughout the labor. Remind yourself of how to do this "Long Deep Breathing" (see page 121).

As I mentioned previously, please do not use the breaths from this book once your cervix is fully dilated and you are pushing the baby out. You will have assistants with you—midwives, doctors and possibly doulas—who will guide you to use other breathing techniques at appropriate times.

FEAR OF LABOR

Something that I have not mentioned until now is tocophobia, or fear of labor. This is a phobic response to the thought of labor and/or going into labor. The result is an avoidance of the subject on any level. Everything that you are learning in this book will help, especially the breathwork in this section, but if you know you have a deep terror of labor, be assured that it is a known phobia and one that can be worked through. Professional help is advised.

BUILDING UP A PRACTICE

The art is to take on these challenging breathwork processes gently. You may want to build up your resilience by increasing your practice time. I suggest starting at around six months pregnant and building up the time over the days. Take on one breath for 30 days, starting at three minutes, and build up from there to five or even eleven minutes.

I know that the work I did for myself in building my endorphin levels and my trust in their ability to reward me was a deciding factor in my two home births. I built up my practice to 11 minutes a day in the last three months of each pregnancy and loved the after-effects each morning. I felt resilient and, over the weeks, that inner sense of self and my own strength grew.

My last thought here is that I absolutely loved both my labors—I know! With each one, once the child was born, I wanted to go through the whole process of birth again. Instantly. My own view of my ability, even now in my sixties, to hold and contain myself and my resilience came through the gift of this work in that time.

TWINS, TRIPLETS AND MORE

It is rare for hospitals to allow a natural birth with twins or multiple births. I am not saying they will not, but the accepted wisdom, for good reason, is that these births will be assisted. I have not taught these specific endorphin-releasing breaths to women bearing twins, triplets or more and suggest trusting the advice of your midwives, doctor or obstetrician with regards to how your labor will be handled. Please do not use this section if you are carrying twins or multiple births.

CLEARING THE HISTORY IN THREE PARTS

This is a three-part breath meditation.

You may notice during your pregnancy that memories come up, long-forgotten stories rise up to be thought about. This can be a time for deep reflection. Some stories are lovely, funny, sparking great memories. Others can be sad or sharp and perhaps it is time to let these go. This series asks, allows, offers the option for this release.

Each section is practiced for 3–5 minutes. The first two are challenging—perfect for building strength and resilience for labor. The last part is Divine, cleansing, washing away old stories and shames, clearing away detritus that is not now wanted as a parent.

Part 1

Suggested music: *"Gajumaru," Yaima.*

Sit beautifully. You can be on the floor or a chair, with wide knees. Notice how this posture lifts the chest and opens the heart center.

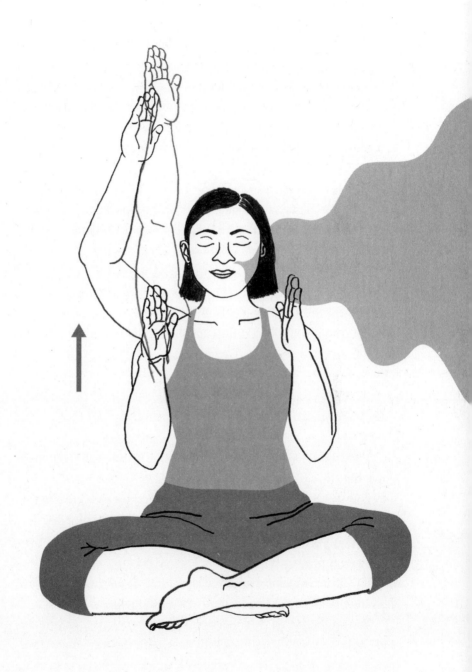

Tuck your elbows in on either side of your ribs, hands facing either side of your face, fingers long and strong.

In this first part, you use your arms and hands as if they were long, sharp swords, rhythmically and alternately pushing up either side. Imagine you are cutting away the memories that you no longer need. See the thoughts as if they lived in a cloud or a fog around and above your head, because this is often how we perceive stressful or unhappy thoughts, as somehow uncontrollable, taking us outside of ourselves.

Your breathing pattern will sort itself out with the movement. There's no need to go super quickly—just shoot each hand up vertically, and then bring it back down to beside your ribs, one after the other. There may be a natural movement, a swaying from side to side, as you do this.

Aim for three minutes. When you have finished, relax your arms down, roll your shoulders and sit in the clear-headed space for two minutes. Notice the endorphins released in support of your effort.

Part 2

Suggested music: *The same as Part 1, or "So Hum," DJ Drez.*

Roll your shoulders, stretch out your legs and rotate your feet, then come back to sitting beautifully.

Put your arms up. If you have high blood pressure, follow the same movement but have your arms out in front of your chest.

Keep the arms straight and hands strong, as before, and criss-cross your arms with the breath, inhaling as the arms open, exhaling as they close. Imagine you are clearing, cleansing, wiping away, polishing the screen of your mind and its thoughts.

Your intention is to be tall and strong, so if you find you are hunching over, sit a little higher. Breathe with the movement, eyes closed, and go with the imagery of clearing, wiping away and shining.

Continue for three minutes. When you have finished, relax your arms down, roll your shoulders and sit in the expansive space for two minutes. Notice the endorphins released in support of your effort.

Part 3

Suggested music: "We Are Love," Jai-Jagdeesh.

Roll your shoulders, stretch out your legs and rotate your feet, then come back to sitting beautifully.

There is an extraordinary magic inherent in this next movement, combined with slow and deep breathing, 5–10 seconds in, 5–10 seconds out.

Close your eyes and see yourself sitting in a beautiful lake of crystal-clear water, up to your waist. There is no discomfort or sense of cold; you are completely comfortable and you know the water is healing.

Reach out in front of you and, with your two hands, scoop up the water. Lift it up above you, raising your face at the same time and then visualize yourself pouring this cool, clear, healing water over your head and face, washing away the hurts, shames and stories.

Over and over, leaning slightly forward on the exhale as you scoop water, and inhaling as you rise up with the hands, wash away all that is no longer needed.

As the process continues, run your fingers through your hair, clearing your face and neck with your hands. Keep going, rhythmically, rocking backward and forward with the compassionate feelings this movement brings. You can include shoulders, breasts, thighs and belly.

This movement is ancient, deep in our DNA. It is the process of forgiveness, absolution and acceptance.

When you have finished, sit and bask in the afterglow of a wonderful breath and movement meditation for clearing the history.

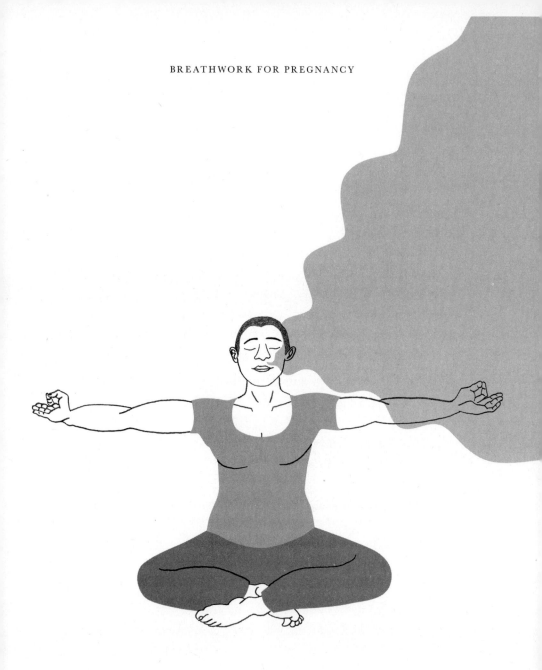

A BREATH TO OPEN THE HEART

Suitable for weeks: Suitable at any point on this journey.
Suggested music: "Beata Viscera," Hilliard Ensemble.

There is a classic *mudra* associated with yoga and meditation called Gyan *mudra*. If I were to say to a ten-year-old child to sit like they were meditating, many of them would instantly sit cross-legged and put the tips of their index fingers to the pads of their thumbs, chest lifted, eyes closed. It is quite a lovely manifestation.

Gyan *mudra* is this classic pose with the hands and it means, in 5,000-year-old Hindu and yogic philosophy, lessons learned with great ease.

Try the *mudra*: bring the index finger and thumb together on each hand, and notice how elegant the hands become. There is a simple beauty inherent in the palms and how the other three fingers naturally find their place.

This is a challenging posture to hold, and here we challenge your perception of all that you are capable of being and doing.

Sit beautifully. You can be on the floor or a chair, with wide knees, back straight. Tilt the chin slightly down. Notice how this posture lifts the chest and opens the heart center. Close your eyes.

Bring your hands into Gyan *mudra*, palms facing each other, fingers vertical, at the center of your chest, elbows wide. Close your eyes and see yourself taking, from the heart center, the negative mind in your left *mudra* and the positive mind in your right *mudra*. Now take your hands out wide either side of you, parallel with the floor, arms straight, palms and *mudra* facing upward. See yourself holding yourself in the strength, presence and stillness of the neutral mind. You are separating yourself from the polarities of the mind and opening the heart.

There is an excellent mantra you can use at this point, one that has come in already. It will help to sustain you in your heart-opening endeavor: *I can, I am.* Bring this into your mind, focus on a slow mental repetition and stay with the posture for as long as you can.

If the discomfort is too much after a minute or so, I suggest that you do not put your arms down as this can trigger a feeling of uselessness. Instead, roll your arms and shoulders over, put your palms down, lean forward, and then open back up again to continue. You may want to start with two minutes and build from there up to eleven minutes. I know! In the first few iterations this may seem unsurmountable but trust me, it is not.

The breath is either "The Straw Breath," inhaling slowly through a rolled tongue and exhaling through the nose (see page 150), or "Long Deep Breathing": 5–10 seconds in, 5–10 seconds out.

You have the breath and the mantra to carry you through.

When you have finished, roll your shoulders, hug them, roll them again and then sit in the delicious waves of endorphins released as the result of your effort for 2–3 minutes. Congratulate yourself for taking apart your self-limiting beliefs and discovering how strong you are.

FINDING STRENGTH AND RESILIENCE

Suitable for weeks: Suitable at any point on this journey.
Suggested music: "Time," Hans Zimmer.

This is a breath technique set with the intention to know your strength.

In playing with all these different breaths you have discovered so many varied ways to breathe. Here is a very unusual breath that asks you to clench your teeth together, pull your lips back and hiss in through the clenched teeth. Then exhale through the nose. Try as you read. This has a strong effect on the vagus nerve and on the tongue and creates a deep inhale.

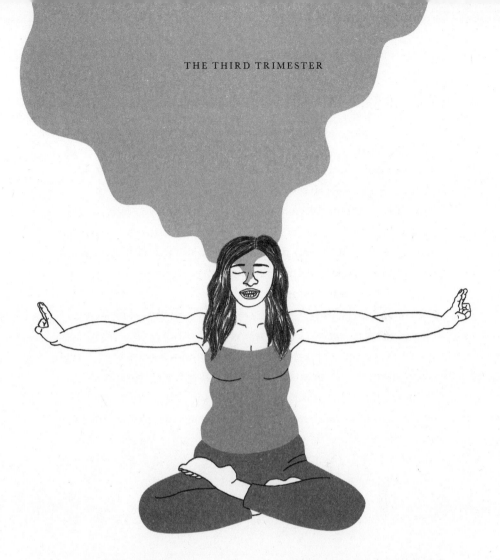

You are also going to have a strong arm posture with another specific *mudra*. Bring your hands up and, keeping the first two fingers tall and locked together, hold down the other two curled fingers with your thumb on the second knuckle on each hand. Try this, too, as you read.

Sit beautifully. You can be on the floor or a chair, with wide knees, back straight. Tilt the chin slightly down. Notice how this posture lifts the chest and opens the heart center.

Using the *mudra* described above, take your arms wide open, parallel to the floor on either side of you, with your palms vertical, the *mudra* facing out. Your arms will form a long line on either side of you, with your hands as vertical as you can make them.

Close your eyes and clench the tips of your teeth together, pull your lips back and hiss in through clenched teeth. Exhale through the nose. Aim for 5–10 seconds in and out.

If the discomfort is too much after a minute or so, I suggest that you do not put your arms down as this can trigger a feeling of uselessness. Instead, roll your arms and shoulders over, turn your palms down and then roll the arms back to continue. You may want to start with two minutes and build from there up to eleven minutes. I know! In the first few iterations this may seem unsurmountable, but trust me, it is not.

When you have finished, roll your shoulders, hug them, roll them again and then sit in the lovely wash of endorphins for 2–3 minutes.

Congratulate yourself for actively taking on finding strength and resilience.

BIRTH TRAUMA

The term "birth trauma" can equally be applied to your experience and to your newborn's. I will avoid listing the possible events that can cause it here.

The traumatic experiences and consequences of birth for the mother can be short or long term. There will be medical assistance in the moment, during birth and for anything that continues to be an issue in the long term.

Trauma—as already explored in earlier chapters, where it has been contextualized as a tall dark history—has a specific effect on the mind–body axis. We know that the major muscles of the pelvis are engaged in the birth process. Alongside any possible tears or incisions, there will be discomfort in stretching out due to stitches and possible lesions. The sympathetic system will be fully engaged, and there may be distressing flashbacks, thought processes and visceral memories of the painful and unexpected physical interventions needed to ensure a safe delivery.

With birth trauma, the amygdala takes off into an outer-world orbit that can feel irretrievable, and perhaps for a few days or weeks, in concert with so many of the new experiences of parenthood, it can be difficult to know what is up and what is down. Where did the peace of the pregnancy go? Can you ever retrieve it?

The stretching chapter does take birth trauma into account to release this physical and emotional overload in the short term. If you have had an episiotomy or a tear in the pelvic floor, this will need time to heal, so the "Standing Stretches" (page 110) will be the most useful until you no longer have stitches. The traumatic response can be held in the body in terms of memories and flashbacks. In this event, "Sufi Grind" (page 100) and "Spinal Flexes" (page 98), both done slowly and kindly, will help to release the intense physical mobilization. If you can allow yourself and those around you time to reset, it will help. This combination of experiences has an intense effect on the mind, body and family members, so do set aside time to release the tension.

If you have flashbacks, an exaggerated startle response, etc., for more than three months, see your doctor. Cognitive behavioral therapy can be effective, as can talking through the birthing process with a mental health professional. Talking to someone trained to listen can assist in diminishing the traumatic responses and create more of a narrative around a shocking event.

Chapter 9

The Fourth Trimester

You open the front door with a huge smile. Held like a sacred scarab, curled in your elbow and nestled against your shoulder, is a delightful little bundle of heaven: your new baby.

"Come in! I am so happy you are here," you say, one arm sweeping wide in a generous invitation to enter.

My gaze follows your hand into the main room. It is a new-parents shambles. A duvet and huge pillows crowd the sofa; an empty water jug, glasses and burp cloths dot the landscape. It is good to see that you are relaxed enough not to be seen as perfect and tidy.

I put the flowers in a vase, the fruit in a bowl and refill the water jug for you. By this time, you are ensconced in warmth and comfort on the sofa and somehow your baby is still asleep.

Herbal tea for you, black tea for me. I move a pile of baby clothes aside and get comfortable.

The invitation to tell me everything opens you up to tears, which glide gently from the sides of your eyes and pool in your ears as you lie back, searching the ceiling. You know how we do visual scanning to see so many different experiences, one after the other.

"It is so great that you came to see me again," you say. "The other side is quite surprising, I feel so … words don't seem to work to describe all the changes, experiences and new realities. I cannot find myself, who I am, yet. It's all moving so fast and I am so exhausted. I felt so beautiful, so abundant, so glorious and magnificent by the last few weeks of pregnancy. Overnight I have become … I

feel, deflated, ugly, fat, sore and I cry so much. Rob has been wonderful, but it is a lot for him too. I am sorry ..."

"Don't apologize for any of this," I say gently. "It is good to cry now, with joy and overwhelm. You will ease everything held inside. They say tears release stress hormones and right now, one week post-labor, the pregnancy hormones are still descending. It is quite usual to cry a lot in the first week."

You nod, sighing with relief, and carefully bring yourself and the tiny girl upright.

The tears continue to drop, plump and glistening, onto the carpet. "Don't get me wrong, I am so happy."

Watching you laughing and crying at the same time, I can feel the huge emotions and tears come to my eyes.

"Shall I hold her so you can tell me how the birth went? What have you called her?"

"Lily ... she is Lily." I love the name.

Now I am the holder of heaven. The perfume of a newborn is so divine, so intoxicating. I breathe in the warmth of Lily's head, and she is relaxed, soft, sleeping and safe.

You dive straight into a sharp memory from the birth and I put my palm up, a silent stop sign. "Slow down. Begin at the point you first knew labor was imminent. When you talk about the stages, in the sequence you experienced them, it helps the brain to process those moments when you felt you were out of control. Can you notice how you went directly to that scary point? Begin again."

You nod and lean forward, elbows on your knees, hands wiping away the tears. I smile as I watch you stretch and roll your shoulders, and this makes you laugh.

"Everything that we did together helped me in such unexpected ways, thank you."

I put my hand on my heart and bow my head in respect. "You took yourself on, you understood the potency of learning to be present, and from the months of stretching and breathwork I can feel how calm Lily is, how she trusts you and can sleep. Well done you, all three of you."

Gently and slowly you talk me through Lily's labor. More tears are shed and there are moments when the memories need to be slowed down, to be explored, moment by moment. By the end of the story you seem tired and yet I can see that this way of processing in detail, in sequence, has created a narrative for you of success and victory, rather than a highlight reel of scary moments.

"It is a heroine's journey to give birth. You have moved through a portal into so many new aspects of both yourself and Rob. I am glad he was there with you. He may be feeling, seeing, remembering the stronger moments too. Does he talk to his friends?"

Rob has been able to go over his version of events, what he saw and felt, how he saw you, it seems, and you are both doing well as new parents.

Lily starts to move and quickly lets us know she is hungry. While you feed her, I make hot soup and more tea.

When feeding time is over, all is calm. "Before I leave I want to show you one last gift in this new phase. It will help you to feel more contained, will facilitate the involution process and keep your kidneys warm, helping you to feel safer. Energetically, the kidneys are said to hold fear and stress, so the warmth is soothing. Did you know it takes 12 hours for the milk to be made? If Lily seems to be uncomfortable after her feed, think back to what you had to eat 12 hours ago."

You are surprised to discover this about breast milk and now, with a quiet baby, you are eager for the gift. "Do you have a six-foot-long wool shawl?" You instantly, and with obvious satisfaction, retrieve one from beneath the snowy duvet.

"In the pregnancy training I run we practice a lost art: belly binding. I will show how to wrap a warm shawl, on the diagonal, around your belly and down to your hips. Belly binding is still practiced routinely in South America and in China. Who knew? I know ...

"Hold the shawl by one corner." This takes a few moments to understand, but you do it, exactly. It is now longer and draped diagonally on the warp and the weft. "Keeping this long diagonal shape, you can notice that it has elasticity if you pull on it." You pull on the shawl and see this is true.

"You want this movement in the binding. Wrap one end around and under your ribs, comfortably tightly, and then keep wrapping it around you down to

the top of your hips. Tuck the end point in under the last bind around your belly."

You stand up and do as asked.

"There! You have bound your belly."

"It feels really good!" you say, moving the bands to cover yourself more completely and tucking it in a little deeper. "It does feel warming, secure, I feel held. I like it, thank you." I check it is not too tight by asking you to sit down. All is good, it seems.

"You can use this on a daily basis for the first few weeks, and it is useful when you find yourself feeling ungrounded or insecure at any time during the rest of your adult life."

Congratulations on the birth of your child. You have been on a mighty and heroic journey through pregnancy, in its three trimesters and, however the labor was for you and your baby, you are now on the other side and building a new series of relationships with your family, motherhood and your body.

Welcome to the fourth trimester. Well done.

The ending of the first three trimesters is the labor process, which can take a quick few hours or many days. Everyone's experience is a different story. There are people who give birth and can lean back into being the epitome of a calm and happy parent. I hope that is you.

It was not me ... and perhaps, in part, that is why I have spent so much of my life working with pregnant women to facilitate, in particular, this postnatal phase.

Having a baby is exhausting—not just the labor, but also the first few months with your newborn. If you think you have been tired before, you have no idea until you give birth. And feed. And don't sleep. It will not just be you, if you are the birthing parent, who feels this. It is easy, as a parent, to feel overwhelmed, hysterical, fearful, fraught and, in this, to find that your significant other is challenged, too.

Rather like walking toward getting married, when all you might think about is what will you wear, our brains don't tend to think beyond labor, particularly with the first child. It can come as a real shock to find yourself in any number of situations in the few hours immediately after birth.

All of a sudden that internalized and deeply embodied growing baby who was with you 24/7, in every moment of thought and feeling, is now outside you. A new person is in your bed, on your lap, in a bassinet beside you and whoever you are partnered with. Do you have any idea what you are supposed to do? Or how to do any of those things? Interesting times.

Exploring the mind and body experience on the other side of labor holds so many possibilities for how you will process the transformation. Each experience is unique and yet there are stages that can be marked in time.

Involution, the process by which the uterus returns to menstruation, takes several weeks, and there is also the release of the lochia, the postnatal fluids. Something no one tells you is that the belly can still appear pregnant for a couple of weeks after delivery. This is due to water retention, muscle memory and uterus size.

The experiences of labor and the postnatal phase can bring attendant physical discomfort for multiple reasons. There can be many things to contend with in the early days and weeks post-birth, such as establishing breastfeeding, getting to grips with the timing of feeds and recovering from perineal bruising or stitches, hemorrhoids, anal fissures and a caesarean, if you've had one. Only you know how you feel in your body and mind.

Nothing will ever be the same again, and that is momentous. For the first few weeks, I strongly suggest keeping yourself in tune with the baby and sleeping whenever they do. Taking time to stretch and breathe will also really help. I promise.

CRYING AND EXHAUSTION

It is quite usual to find yourself crying for around four days after birth, the tears seemingly unstoppable. This is a natural part of the hormonal changes occurring within you. The gestational hormones are plummeting, and crying is one way that certain hormones leave the body. Crying in the first few days after delivery, whatever form this took, is absolutely normal. Even though it may not feel great and can contribute to the sensations of helplessness and so much being unknown, new and different, it is in how we respond to the crying that we create suffering for ourselves.

If your birth experience was traumatic and you now understand what this means for the mind and body, these tears can be from relief, pain and the discomfort of tears and stitches, or post-traumatic memories, triggering overwhelm. Again, this is all normal, but if you do find it is going on for longer than expected, it is advisable to talk with your midwife or health professional.

Exhaustion is another challenging experience, both physically and mentally, but it is also normal. My own experience was that I had no idea of real exhaustion until the first few months of the postnatal phase.

Stretching will help all round, but remember that in the first weeks after delivery your pelvis will still be loose from the relaxin wearing off, so take care not to overstretch.

POSTNATAL STRETCHING

Stretching changes in the postnatal phase and certain movements that were impossible before will now be available to you.

There is no rush to sit cross-legged, if that is your goal, or to be able to sit and practice your stretches and breaths with the same calm that you may have been able to achieve in pregnancy. (If you have previous children around you, then you will be well versed in interruptions.) This time with the new child is important for the bonding process and you will have bed rest and feeding hours in which to breathe consciously.

You do not have to be a superhero in the first few weeks. If you feel that you *should* keep up a regular practice, this will only add to the overwhelm. When your baby is asleep, certainly in the first three months, you should sleep too! Please don't take this time to try to achieve postnatal perfection.

The art of stretching early in the postnatal phase is to take it gently, slowly and kindly.

When you allow the mind to dwell on the stinging or pulling sensations, the sore places in your body, alongside whatever resistance there may be to how the postpartum process is going, it is easy to spiral into feelings that negate your sense of self.

Pain, for whatever reason, is unpleasant, and you can alleviate much of it by slowing down and putting your mind to a task. Take over the amygdala (see Chapter 2) and soften your reactivity. To consciously breathe is to take a step away and soothe the self.

Perhaps you had to have an episiotomy. Simple steps like stretching the front of the body before having a pee, taking a few deep inhales through tight lips and exhaling through the nose will release the contracted pelvic floor, which may be behind the dreaded stinging feeling.

When you have sore nipples and are facing *another* feed, the internal sense of contraction can be released consciously and the let-down will happen, the attunement will be made easier.

Stretch in bed prior to and after feeding to reset the mind and clear the lymph. Your baby will enjoy being beside you, basking in the relaxation, interrupting your flow, wanting to be fed. How you respond to this is, as ever, a choice.

In stretching you will notice how cramped and rolled forward the shoulders can feel. Long periods of having your arms out in front of you and curved around the baby will affect posture, specifically in the back and between the shoulder blades. There are props to help with releasing these tensions (see page 10).

BREATHWORK AND THE POSTNATAL PHASE

Please do not use these breathing techniques while pregnant. At all.

You will know the breaths that you like by now from Chapter 5, and you can use them as and when you want the bliss of the breath, or when you are overwhelmed and perhaps in another cycle of adjusting to the many changes continually coming into your new reality.

Recognizing the power of conscious breathwork and, in that, coming to this section of the book is a continuing journey into better attachment, attunement and an ever-evolving ability to hold yourself in the face of challenging times as life unfurls in front of you.

Once you have given birth, it is important to wait a minimum of six weeks before learning the techniques here. This is because it takes this long for the womb to involute (see page 208). It is not advisable to interrupt this process with strong breathwork. Please, even if you are longing to get on with regaining your strength, do wait for your body to settle out of the immediate after-effects of the birth. Starting to belly pump—"Breath of Fire" (page 214)—too early, is not advisable. To wait for the body to settle is to be kind and gentle to yourself.

All the breathwork in Chapter 5 is still available to you at this time, and there are very different experiences to be had in trying breaths that you found uncomfortable in pregnancy.

I am also aware, based on many years of teaching pre- and postnatal breathwork, that there can be a rush, a pressure, perhaps a sense of need not only to get back to life as you may have known it, but also to lose some of the weight gained in pregnancy. Social media is flooded with images of women with a postnatal six-pack, and lucky them. For some, it is their metabolism that allows this vision of recovery perfection, but most of them are not actually filming themselves in the first few months of having a new baby. We are all built differently, we process each individual pregnancy in a new way, and in a book about finding calm through managing how you think and feel, perhaps recognize that it is important to take some time—weeks or months—to adapt and adjust to all the changes in your daily reality. You do not need to be perfect, so cut yourself some slack. Making a baby is monumental work.

Your body may not be close to the perfection that you feel you deserve for such an extraordinary act of creation, and this is its own challenge. You will recover, on all fronts, and may even decide to have another child at some point, but leave that for now—just be kind to yourself, to the baby.

In this postnatal phase, your breathwork options include work to bring heat back into the body. Think about the momentous work that your body has done for nine months, creating a child from a single egg (maybe two) and sperm. This creative feat is a fiery energy. In a sense, it is possibly the biggest act of creativity you could ever be part of. You will notice, when you relax in the exhaustion and bliss of the postpartum phase, that if you put your hand on your belly, it is cold. All the fiery energy that the Chinese call your *chi* is now outside your body, in the child. Bringing fire back into your own body, through breathwork, will really help you regain your sense of self, strength and energy.

WHEN YOUR CHILD IS IN ICU

To have a child in the intensive care unit (ICU) is terrifying and stressful in equal measure. Premature birth and delivery issues can be the cause of this forced separation, which may also mean that you, too, are dealing with all manner of personal, traumatic and internal recovery issues. If you have a partner, there is the added inter-relational stress, and going home at night, leaving the baby alone, is profoundly difficult.

I have experienced having a child in the ICU and I am aware of how that felt for me. All I could do, in my sense of utter helplessness and fear, was to stretch and take time to breathe. To sit, despite my madly scavenging mind playing out every disaster, and keep on softening, releasing. Holding and containing myself gave me the real ability to be utterly present when I was in the ICU ward.

I did use prayer in these moments. That may or may not be something you believe in, but the prayer of the mother is said to be one of the most potent.

In these times, doing breathwork together, and in the presence of your baby, can be healing and bonding for both you and your partner. Coming together to soften, to reset and to take time for the self-healing process for you as a couple is a potent act of parenting. If you are able to touch your baby in that calm and gentle space, when you have stretched and soothed yourselves, they will be responsive to this hormonal and energetic shift. They will be aware that you are better attuned. It will soothe them, too.

You will know which breath to suggest and show your partner. You will have a sacred space in which to bond in love and stillness, to stand down for a few minutes from the stresses of your daily routine. Allow recovery time for you, for a body that has been through an intense process and is now transforming again.

If you are expressing milk for your child, then after these releasing sessions it will be easier to let down the milk.

BREATH OF FIRE

You are invited, in this first exercise, to begin to learn "Breath of Fire."

"To begin to learn"—notice these particular four words. You will learn how to breathe in this way. As with several of the other breaths you have made friends with, "Breath of Fire" is an ancient yogic technique and it takes time to master. It is a breath technique that you *learn* how to do. It is a breath that asks you to pump your belly, thus moving the huge muscle that is your diaphragm up and down using muscles you may never have used before.

"Breath of Fire" comes to the fore now because, as we've just covered, the process of gestation and birth has literally removed fire energy, or *chi*, from your body. This fire energy is now in your baby. You are going to learn to breathe in a way that reignites the embers in your navel area, bringing heat and a sense of vitality into your being. This way of breathing also affects your mind, body, oxygen levels and hormone levels, plus it strengthens and tones the stomach muscles. It is a stimulating, energetic breath.

"Breath of Fire" massages the intestines, which relaxes the vagus nerve and releases serotonin into the body and brain (see pages 31 and 56). Released when the system is relaxed and gentle, serotonin facilitates stillness and presence. You are going to take on a vigorous breathwork practice to bask in very interesting, different states of stillness as a reward for the effort expended.

The potency of this technique is such that it does affect menstruation. It will make the blood flow stronger on the first two days, and so will move the period more quickly through your body. It is up to you if you want this or not. "Breath of Fire" is a magical and generating breath that will also increase your fertility, if that is what you want, later down the line.

You have so far used breathwork to take over the unconscious aspect of the breathing mechanism by releasing and stretching the diaphragm, thereby taking yourself into the parasympathetic system (see page 52). "Breath of Fire" is an ancient yogic technique that invites a fast, rhythmic pumping, forcing the diaphragm to contract and empty the lungs as it pushes up. This breathing technique asks you to suspend the natural breathing mechanism and take over the diaphragm. The inhale is silent; there is no sound. You release the muscles to let the diaphragm drop, thus automatically inhaling. You will go into your whole physicality and, by the action of pumping, say to the system, *You're mine, you're mine, you're mine*, over and over.

Breath of Fire is different from, and often confused with, another practice known as *bhastrika*, or bellows breath, which involves a forceful exhale *and* a forceful inhale: dragging air in, forcefully pushing air out and hearing your breath both ways. This is *not* what we are working toward in learning "Breath of Fire."

Given that such extraordinary transformations have happened to your stomach muscles over the weeks of pregnancy, and that you have likely done very little core exercise until now, other than lifting and carrying your baby and whatever tasks you have taken on in your daily reality, this tightening of the belly area will be a new physical experience.

It does sound complicated, but getting started requires simple focus on a few main points.

Getting started

To get the most out of the initial learning, sit wide-kneed, with elbows locked, chest lifted. Open your mouth and quickly tighten your stomach muscles to force the air out of the lungs. There is a sound in the throat as this happens, like a dog panting in the heat of a summer's day. The inhale has no sound, you just release and drop the tightened stomach muscles, thus relaxing the diaphragm down again and thereby inhaling.

Start slowly, try a few times and make sure that as you exhale forcefully, your belly goes in, not out! Then move onto ten rhythmic exhales, getting used to the dropping sensation to achieve a silent inhale. If you lose the rhythm, slow right down and gradually speed up again.

Be aware of your facial muscles as you do this. It is counter-intuitive and yet oh so easy to frown. Try to keep your face calm. We are taking time here to establish good technique and avoid the bad habits that can easily be established with this breath.

Music really does work well for this breath, and I will suggest fast tracks for each of the different Breath of Fire styles to come. Good music with a beat makes it easier to maintain a well-paced rhythm.

Breath of Fire with the mouth open

Suggested music: *"Yr Love," Holy Other.*

This is the simplest way to learn and become familiar with the rhythmic diaphragmatic pump and release required for this breathing style.

When you do Breath of Fire with the mouth open, the sensation is actually cooling and calming, so the name can feel like a misnomer, a distraction—yet it still has the same benefits of igniting fire and generating energy, as well as cooling the "emotional body."

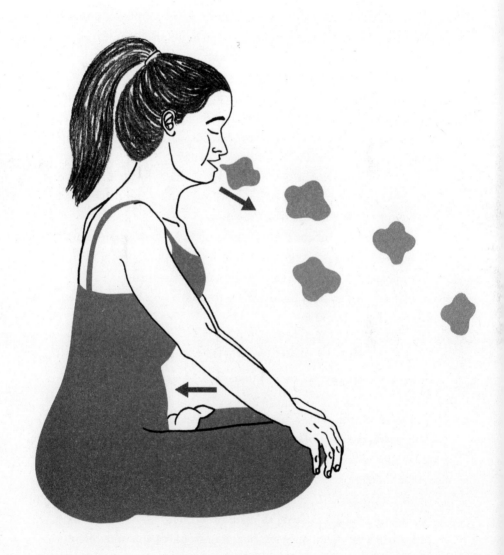

Sit beautifully. You can be on the floor or a chair, with wide knees, back straight. Tilt the chin slightly down. Notice how this posture lifts the chest and opens the heart center. You can do Gyan *mudra* or not, it is up to you.

Close your eyes and open your mouth. Keep your facial muscles relaxed and aim to keep your knees still. Do not use them to propel the breath out by lifting with each pump.

Set a timer for three minutes.

Start the music, if you are using any, and begin the rhythmic, strong exhale, alternating with the silent dropping of the diaphragm to inhale. If you lose the rhythm, slow down and build back up again. Continue in this way for three minutes.

When you have finished, take a deep inhale through the nose and hold the breath while pulling and tightening the pelvic floor and diaphragm, chin tilted slightly down.

Hold for 3–5 seconds. You may need to keep retightening the pelvic floor during this time and that is OK. Again, it is a muscle that may not have had much strengthening post-birth.

Sit still, oh so still, filled with serotonin and oxygen, embers fired up, for 2–3 minutes.

Breath of Fire with the tongue out

Suggested music: *"Orango" (instrumental), Niju.*

You have played with a breath-and-tongue combination before. This particular style of rapid, pumping breath requires the tongue to be pushed far out, not a little kitten tongue. This maintains a pull on the vagus nerve, via the tongue, and combines with the diaphragmatic pumping.

There is an added layer of coolness brought about by this style of breath. The effect, once finished, is quite particular and different again to the previous open-mouthed style.

Sit beautifully. You can be on the floor or a chair, with wide knees, back straight. Tilt the chin slightly down. Notice how this

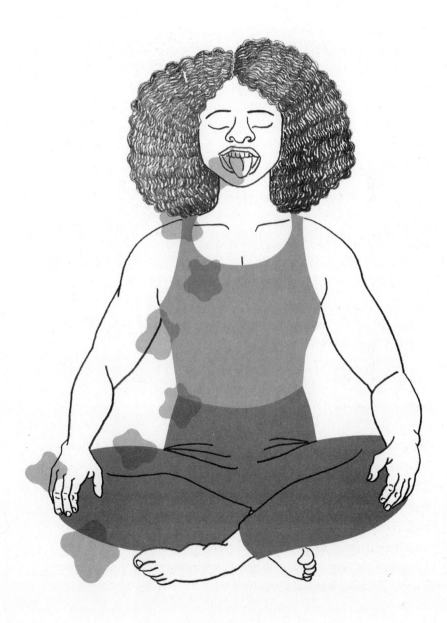

posture lifts the chest and opens the heart center. You can do Gyan *mudra* or not, it is up to you.

Close your eyes and open your mouth, pushing your tongue far out. Do not hold the tongue with your teeth, just stick it out. Keep your facial muscles relaxed and notice how easy it is to smile like this. Aim to keep your knees still; do not use them to propel the breath out by lifting with each pump.

Set a timer for three minutes.

Start the music, if you are using any, and begin the rhythmic, strong exhale, alternating with the silent dropping of the diaphragm to inhale. If you lose the rhythm, slow down and build back up again. The tongue should stay out throughout unless you need to swallow or lubricate. Continue in this way for three minutes.

When you have finished, bring the tongue in and take a deep inhale through the nose, then hold the breath while pulling and tightening the pelvic floor and diaphragm, chin tilted slightly down. Hold for 3–5 seconds. You may need to keep retightening the pelvic floor during this time and that is OK. Again, it is a muscle that may not have had much strengthening post-birth.

Sit still with the sensation of vibrant energy in the body for 2–3 minutes. Try to maintain the smile!

Breath of Fire with the mouth closed

Suggested music: *"Meditation," Turu Anasi.*

This is perhaps the most traditional way of practicing Breath of Fire and it is generally seen as the most heating. The breath is entirely done through the nose. All the same awareness applies, including keeping the face relaxed, perhaps with a small smile, and using a silent inhale. It is a different experience in the practice and in the post-breath stillness.

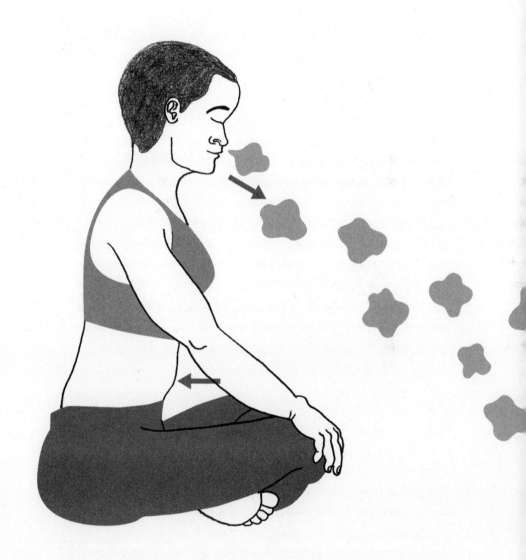

Sit beautifully. You can be on the floor or a chair, with wide knees, back straight. Tilt the chin slightly down. Notice how this posture lifts the chest and opens the heart center. You can do Gyan *mudra* or not, it is up to you.

Close your eyes. Keep your facial muscles relaxed and aim to keep your knees still. Do not use them to propel the breath out by lifting with each pump.

Set a timer for three minutes.

Start the music, if you are using any, and begin the rhythmic, strong exhale, alternating with the silent dropping of the diaphragm to inhale through the nose. If you lose the rhythm, slow down and build back up again. If you cannot refind the rhythm, go back to open-mouthed breathing for a few rounds and then close the mouth again. Continue in this way for three minutes.

When you have finished, take a deep inhale through the nose and hold the breath while pulling and tightening the pelvic floor and diaphragm, chin tilted slightly down.

Hold for 3–5 seconds. You may need to keep retightening the pelvic floor during this time and that is OK. Again, it is a muscle that may not have had much strengthening post-birth.

Sit still, silent, utterly still, with no mind and no breath at all for as long as this expansive state lasts, and then breathe gently for 2–3 minutes.

BREATHS AND BABY FEEDING

Feeds are a vastly time-consuming part of early parenting, whether you're breast- or bottle-feeding, using a combination of the two, or expressing.

Some babies and parents find it easy and the latch is perfect from the first moment. Others, myself included, feel as though we are going into battle with our boobs, the bottle and the baby! This experience only ends up winding itself up into all manner of unpleasant thoughts about ourselves, feelings of being a bad parent and not doing it right, and comparison to others. This in turn becomes stressful for the baby.

Conscious breathing really can be amazing now. It is in sitting and feeding—with the bottle or the breast, sometimes for extended periods, many times a day—that you can use calming breaths to land yourself into presence. This state has a profound effect on everyone around you, particularly the baby, as well as soothing your own fractious thoughts and feelings.

Take a moment to roll your shoulders and stretch up, releasing any premade decisions about how this time will be, letting go of any gearing up for discomfort you may have done. You know now that you can change how you show up for this really important time. Remember the oxytocin and the attunement that you can bring to this meeting of you and your baby, every time, over and over.

Use breaths that feel gentle and calming. You will know which ones these are for you by now. Avoid noisy breaths that have tight-lipped inhales and let the breath soften you, the baby and anyone in your vicinity.

In terms of breathing posture, it tends to be best if you can sit up, but for now, when feeding, do whatever feels right and comfortable for you.

Do stretch the back, arms and front of the chest after a feed, too, releasing tension from the long and contracted hold.

BREASTFEEDING WITHOUT BIRTHING

If the non-childbearing parent in a same-sex couple is choosing to stimulate breast milk to share in the feeding, this is a commitment to time, patience and a regular process of breast manipulation for 20 minutes every 3 hours, 24 hours a day. This is another opportunity to breathe together, to share the experiences of gestation via their swelling, painful and changing breasts. You do not need or may not even want to be back to back, as this is a physical process, but it can ease the discomfort, isolation and stress over the weeks leading up to the birth to allow this to be a chosen time to practice together.

CREATING A PERSONAL PRACTICE

A personal mantra, and one that I often tell myself as I feel thoughts and feelings contract within me, is: *Step away, beautiful person, and give yourself and everyone around you a break.*

The postnatal phase is generally considered to be 4–6 weeks in terms of involution, establishing breastfeeding and physically recovering from an episiotomy. What is not spoken aloud, but must be named, is that it takes two years to recover from a pregnancy.

I have no intention of being the harbinger of doom on any level. I am aware that reading that sentence could seem deflating, but my intention is to bring awareness and compassion to a complex process for the growing baby, your partnership and you as the evolving mother or primary carer.

Humans are born utterly vulnerable, more so than any other mammal on the planet. Think of the biggest mammals—elephants, giraffes, horses; they can all stand to suckle within a couple of hours of birth. We have had to compromise in our evolutionary development to accommodate our very large brains, and extreme vulnerability for an extended period is the price. It is generally the mother who pays for this through her physical sacrifice in terms of gestation, carrying, caring, feeding and nurturing.

You probably know all this and are wondering why I've included it in a piece about personal practice.

Personal practice means committing to a daily routine of time and space that is sacred and sacrosanct—two very beautiful words.

Sacred is the beauty of the time and space, what you choose to do in that chosen space, the mat, the stretches and breathwork. You consciously build a relationship with yourself, knowing that this has a positive impact on your sense of self, your relationships, your environment and your offspring.

Sacrosanct means that this is a commitment you make that is important to you—you stand by it, you choose to take the time and space, it is inviolate.

Come back, now, to the two years that it takes to recover from pregnancy. In my decades of teaching, personal experience and working with mothers, parents, yoga and breathwork, I have witnessed many people feel useless for being unable to commit to a daily practice in these first two years, for good reason. It is impossible to be good, perfect, carve out time and just sit breathing as the laundry piles up, the kids cry and the next meal waits to be made.

At the time of writing, I have been working with my own practice for over 30 years. When I started, my own mind–body axis had been put out of kilter by early experiences and, once clean and sober, I understood that it was entirely up to me to actively change how I felt and reacted, rather than demanding or expecting someone else to do it for me.

As I wrote in the early pages, I have had two children since I took myself on. I so wanted, after the first child, to return to my sacrosanct daily practice, but I could not for multiple reasons. I learned a valuable lesson that I would like to share with you.

During these two years you can stretch in bed, before a shower or on the carpet while the kids are playing. You can breathe while watching football or folding the laundry. Remember that you can change how you feel and you can commit to doing this in some way each day.

Create the sacred and the sacrosanct by having a lovely bath, making delicious cupcakes, going out for a picnic, picking meadow flowers, singing while you wash up, dancing with your baby in your arms, watching the sun set each evening, lighting candles on the dinner table, eating with your family as often as you possibly can. Choose to take on acts of kindness and presence as your personal daily practice.

There are many different ways to mark and notice the sacred and the sacrosanct. When you feel as though you have come through those first two years, you may well be ready to have another child, or you can take time and space to commit to a daily practice on the mat. By then, everything that has already been established in the small and precious moments you choose to make each day will still be there.

TO A SINGLE OR LONELY PARENT

If you are a single or lonely parent, for any number of reasons, this time is difficult. I do not wish to presume that you are incapable on any level. Single parenting is, for some, a choice that has been thought through. Partners can also be absent, physically and emotionally, for extended periods of time. I hope you have friends, family and good support around you.

The postnatal phase is, by its very nature, a time of transformation, and as a single mother, so much is up to you and only you. This includes recovery time for your body, the complex transformation from being pregnant to being a mother, and the hours spent feeding and watching your life around you in terms of simple daily tasks like laundry, managing a stroller and shopping, which can feel almost herculean.

As a single parent there can be little or no relief, a rare sharing of responsibility. If you have people coming in to assist you in various ways, there can be an added burden of perceived debt and a need to push back to a semblance of normality as quickly as possible. These feelings easily become too complex to hold and process. Isolation is then magnified and the loneliness can be unbearable.

It may be that you have already had children, in which case the burden can weigh even more heavily upon you.

Remind yourself, when you feel lost, angry or as though your brain has become soup through lack of sleep and too much to do, that you have so many tools available to you from Chapters 4 and 5. You can stretch out stress and frustration and you can breathe consciously to allow for a sense of presence to reappear. With all you have now learned about breathwork and stretching, you could create a small group who come together to stretch and breathe.

If you notice your mood is sinking, do reach out to your health professionals to be referred to a counselor. Help and support are out there for you.

Becoming a Conscious Parent

"Can I tell you a story? It is a curious one and you may, at the end, think I am as crazy as a box of frogs. But you may also begin to see why you are the center of the universe, the axis mundi, *now you are a parent. My hope is that in all the work we have done together, an awareness will emerge for you about how much more there is to you, to life and the future than you may allow for, see or experience now."*

"Oh, yes!" you say. "I love a story. Can we do it by candlelight?"

"Yes!" I light three candles and turn off the lights.

"Then I will begin. As you know, I am a woman and I have short hair. An odd start, but bear with me here. This morning I went to the barber. Yes, I go to a barber, as they do a better cut, and Abdul from Kurdistan is a master cutter. He started training at 14 and is now in his early forties.

"When I sit in the chair for this delightful experience, I aim to be completely relaxed, calm, but still present and gentle. I respect his work and my time. Once the haircut nears perfection, he uses an old-fashioned cut-throat razor to create a perfect edge to the cut.

"As he uses this sharp blade around my ear, and at the sides and back of my neck, I am keenly aware that I know this feeling deep in my bones, from so many other rounds on this mortal coil. I have sat in a barber's chair in so many other lives, it is in my muscle memory that I move in a way that assists his razor. The feeling is always slightly startling. I know that it is my state of total presence to his work that allows this memory to rise up.

"You are so still, chin on your hands, looking up at me in the candlelight.
"Oh! I love this story! Tell me more."

"I remember when I first started to train as a doula—a person who is there for the mother during labor—that people strongly suggested to me that I should train to be a midwife. I remember sitting with this notion and thinking it through in quiet stillness. It evolved into a curious sensation, like a memory in my DNA from long, long ago. In that state of presence I knew, absolutely, that I had facilitated thousands of births in my many lives, and that I was not going to be a midwife again. I wanted to take a different path."

"Ah ..." you sigh. "I think I understand what you are saying, but keep going. I could listen to this story all night. Go on ..."

"In the nineties I was traveling around India by train. It was utterly excellent and rather eccentric. There were no mobile phones, cameras used film, the internet was in its earliest dial-up form, you had to prebook an international call and tourists relied on Lonely Planet *guides—tomes that listed all the places you could stay.*

"Arriving in the very center of India, at a town called Khajuraho, which is famous for its intricately carved temples, I decided to stay at Yogi Lodge as The Lovely Planet Guide, *as it was known by locals, reported that the yogi who ran it was a seer and a psychic. I arrived with my rucksack and stood in the reception, waiting to get a room. The yogi saw me and walked straight up to me.*

"'You were a boat woman in Greece, ferrying people between the islands, in one of your lives,' he said. 'You drowned in a storm carrying seven people. Everyone died. You have, so far in this life, met four of these people. And earlier in your incarnations you were a seagull.' He walked off and I was open-mouthed with amazement.

"You see, I have a mortal terror of the sea, so his words made sense to me. I could remember the storm, in that moment, and even now as I tell you.

"And I love, adore all birds, but particularly seagulls. I watch them flying, circling, fighting for food scraps, and I know, absolutely, deep in my DNA, how that feels—to fly, to soar, to travel miles and miles over the sea. I know.

"Are you still awake?" I whisper, and you raise your head and say, "Absolutely. I want to know everything."

I could keep going, telling you so many stories like this, but I prefer to return to you now.

"One of the most beautiful flowers I have ever seen was a cream peony with hundreds of petals and a deep red center, in full bloom, open to the morning sunlight, still and stunning.

"And I know, deep, deep in my heart, that I too was that flower that is now on the cover of this book. In its absolute perfection that flower was in love with, and part of, the perfection of the universe.

"Axis mundi is the Latin term that describes the axis of the Earth between the celestial poles. Stay with me here. This is the macrocosm, the big, zoomed-out picture of the world, the cosmos, if you will, with the Earth at the center. In this expanded, expansive view, everything is perfect, held in silent stillness, unfolding in perfect order, for millions of years.

"If we zoom in, we have the microcosm: you, the parent, at the center of this world, your world, your reality.

"This flower was, I was, the axis mundi, the center of the universe. You are now, too. You are in one of the most creative and perfect states of being: raising a child.

"If you feel small and helpless in the face of all that swirls around you, personally and globally, know that you are not alone. You have agency. You are now a different person on so many levels. One person can be an instrument for massive change in all realms. As a mother, as a parent, your microcosmic part in the macrocosm is potent.

"As the 14th Dalai Lama said: 'If you think you are too small to make a difference, try spending the night with a mosquito.'"

Let us take a moment and pause. It is quite possible that a lot is bubbling up for you in response to all that you have read in these pages.

We stand, all of us, at a pivotal time in history/herstory. Events are unfolding, seemingly helplessly, around humanity. And you are now a parent. You know the responsibility you bear, and it is not a trifling one.

My main goal in this book has been for you to be a conscious parent, and you have the learning and tools in your hands right now. You can take steps so that your own story will not negatively affect how you parent.

Throughout pregnancy and into the postnatal period, you have been able to share this ability to manage and hold your emotional being with the next generation. That is the amazing gift of all we have done together. This is work that you do for yourself, and that your children, your family and all around you can benefit from for the rest of your lives.

Conscious parenting is not about being perfect. There is a terrible cultural imperative to be a perfect mother, a perfect parent, which, as we have explored, does not actually exist. If nobody has told you that, it's a bit of a life-changing awakening.

But what you can become—and this is really potent—is a *good enough* parent. And the only person who will allow you to be good enough is you. Nobody else gives you permission.

The combination of breathwork and stretching that we've explored throughout these pages is, I promise with my hand on my steadfast heart, the fastest way to find presence, calm and the glorious expanse of *right here, right now.* If you remember, this is the landscape we are heading to, longing for, between the *pain of the past and fear of the future.* It is in this expanse that we can land into being conscious parents.

Certainly, if this is your first child, this is a rare chance to learn to attune, to hold agency.

As I hope you've come to understand, you are not stuck in your anxiety, your story, your fears or your rages, be they internal or external. You can change how you think and feel. You are not tainted or cursed forever with reactive behaviors, endlessly repeating your past. As you've played with breath and as you've moved through the book, you've learned that it is through the body that we can change the mind.

In learning and applying these skills we can begin, person by person, parent by parent, to make huge changes around us and for the future of those we raise.

In this vast place, we learn to attune, have agency, show our responses rather than our reactivity, hold difficult feelings—be they anger, fear, shame or betrayal—and process them, to find an adult answer or way through. We can take ourselves out of the relentless cycle of victim, persecutor and rescuer, into a place where we, our partners and our children feel safe, nurtured, boundaried and respected.

It has been a pleasure to be beside you in this extraordinary time.

FURTHER READING

100 Things We've Lost to the Internet, Pamela Paul (Random House, Inc., 2021)

Digital Minimalism, Cal Newport (Penguin Business, 2020)

Freedom from the Known, Jiddu Krishnamurti (Rider, 2010)

Full Catastrophe Living, Jon Kabat-Zinn (Piatkus, 2013)

How Emotions Are Made, Lisa Feldman Barrett (Pan, 2018)

Pelvic Liberation, Leslie Howard (Leslie Howard Yoga, 2017)

Rewriting the Rules, Meg-John Barker (Routledge, 2018)

Savage Grace, Andrew Harvey and Carolyn Baker (iUniverse, 2017)

Spiritual Midwifery, Ina May Gaskin (Book Publishing Company, 2002)

The Artist's Way, Julia Cameron (Souvenir Press, 2020)

The Body Keeps the Score, Bessel van der Kolk (Penguin, 2015)

The Continuum Concept, Jean Liedloff (Penguin, 1989)

The Courage to Be Disliked, Ichiro Kishimi and Fumitake Koga (Allen & Unwin, 2019)

The Dance of Anger, Harriet G. Lerner (Element Books, 2004)

The Fourth Trimester, Kimberly Ann Johnson (Shambhala, 2017)

The Functions of the Orgasms, Michel Odent (Pinter & Martin Ltd, 2009)

Why We Sleep, Matthew Walker (Penguin, 2018)

ACKNOWLEDGMENTS

Louis and Isadora, I am so happy that you know who you are.

Bernd Leygraf, consultant psychotherapist,
human being, priest, teacher and fellow traveler.

Satya Kaur and Elena O'Keefe, for all the years of
teaching and learning we experienced together.

Sara-Jayne Edwards, for unwavering support and research.

Sophie Budden, for ruthless readings
and early morning encouragement.

Jane Graham-Maw, my literary agent.

Julia Kellaway, for a wonderful edit—thank you.

All at Vermilion, thank you for believing in this project.

INDEX

ABOUT THE AUTHOR

Carolyn Cowan is a London-based psychotherapist, and yoga and breathwork teacher. She has spent more than 20 years specializing in psychosexual therapy, trauma and relationships, and working with pre- and postnatal clients.

For more information, visit carolyncowan.com.